"Look out cancer! Here comes COURAGE—armed with unorthodox humor, brilliant rage, and remarkable, unshakable faith in God. A stunning memoir of deep emotions, rarely shared in hushed tones—much less bold print. An eye-opening read for women with or without breast cancer, the medical world, clergy—and each of us who care so deeply about those battling the ghastly disease."

– Marion Bond West,
Author/Contributing Editor, *Guideposts*

"I couldn't put this book down—many passages to underline and revisit. Not just for women diagnosed with a serious illness. A must-read for any woman who has had a breast or gynecological exam by a male physician. Even in segments, excerpts from this provocative, detailed account of the unmentionables, the intimacy, the lust, the anger, the hopelessness, the resilience and lack of it, the grief, the humor, love, and mystery, and the healing power of authentic relationships between doctors and patients warrant consideration and discussion. Absolutely required reading for practicing physicians—and those in training."

–Sandra L. Bertman,
PhD, FT

"I honor Connie Titus for seeking to put into writing her own walk of faith during an extraordinary time in her life. Records of this kind inevitably bless not only the people who are in a comparable situation but also other sensitive persons who project themselves into the story and who find their own faith undergirded for their own particular problems."

– Dr. J. Ellsworth Kalas
President, Asbury Theological Seminary

Her Doctor Prescribes

Dancing
at Daybreak

Jan 2009

To Nancy,
May God bless
your reading and
understanding of
my words.
(Choose Life
(Deut. 30: 19-20)

Connie

Her Doctor Prescribes

Dancing at Daybreak

Connie
Thompson
Titus

Lively Doctor-Patient Interactions

TATE PUBLISHING & *Enterprises*

Published by Tate Publishing & Enterprises, LLC
127 E. Trade Center Terrace | Mustang, Oklahoma 73064 USA
1.888.361.9473 | www.tatepublishing.com

Tate Publishing is committed to excellence in the publishing industry. The company reflects
the philosophy established by the founders, based on Psalm 68:11,
"The Lord gave the word and great was the company of those who published it."

Published in the United States of America
ISBN:978-1-60604-138-3
1. Christian Inspiration: Motivational: Biography & Autobiography
2. Medical: Oncology: Breast Cancer
08.12.05

Dedication

I dedicate my work
to all who turn these pages.

May I coax you
to relish life
and dance a little jig
of your own.

ct

Table of Contents

Foreword

"To enjoy good health, first be sick."
Brother Giles, *The Little Flowers of Francis*

Connie Beth Thompson Titus came into my life more than ten years ago. Diagnosed with incurable inflammatory breast cancer, she sought my oncologic opinion. The last decade of our relationship, seen through the eyes of this wondrous cancer survivor, is what is written on these supple pages between two covers. You will envision and experience empowerment, destiny, love, courage, humor, inspiration, coping, transformation, and the ability and permission to truly live. Connie's spirit and determination epitomizes the embodiment of what living with cancer is all about.

In this series of letters, Connie gives too much credit to my leadership and counsel. We both know that her being able to survive is the direct result of her will to live and her acceptance of vast therapeutic options, both conventional and alternative. This book and the writings herein are a true testimony of the restorative and beneficial role of hope combined with the unrelenting audacity of her heroism.

I believe my greatest input in watching this magical miracle unfold was the encouragement I gave her to use her unbelievable literary talent to write this book. I revel in the awe of it all.

Connie, thank you for the honor of allowing me to be part of your healing and thank you for being part of my learning some of life's complex enterprises. Keep *Dancing at Daybreak*!

"I will face my fear. I will permit it to pass over me and through me. Where the fear has gone, there will be nothing. Only I will remain."

Frank Herbert
The Dune Chronicles, Book 1.

—Alan S. Collin, M.D.

Preface

Dear Reader:

The same doctor has been meeting me in Exam Room #3, usually on Tuesdays, for ten years and counting. Do we run out of new things to say to each other? No. Office visits resemble variety shows. My unusual medical history sets the stage, dancing with disease is choreographed, roles reverse between the professional and the amateur, and doctor-patient perspectives either mesh nicely or clash in heated debate. Life is made up along the way. Whatever the scene, our conversations are quite colorful.

You hold a collection of intimate letters written to my oncologist (cancer doctor). These letters replay our Tuesday office visits. Discussions, decisions, and passages through hard places are recorded in an easy-to-read, non-scientific storybook. This is a work of fancy; a work of serious faith. Much of my book is funny. My love for writing draws from rich experience to offer a loose-leaf understanding of oncology. The clinic door is wide open. Come on in.

For medical or nursing students contemplating oncology as your specialty, please take *Dancing at Daybreak* on a trial run. Newly-diagnosed or long-time survivors and all your fearful caregivers, read about zany behavior that will make your thoughts and actions seem normal. Inflammatory Breast Carcinoma sisters, look beyond the predictions of this rare strain and live with zest. Clinicians and counselors, are you weary? I say enter into relationships with your patients/clients. Their reciprocal love and guidance can perk up your practice. To innocent bystanders, this book may change your view of diseased people and men in white coats from here on out.

Speaking of perspectives, in September 2003, I was honored to participate in a day-long Patient Perspective Symposium. To me, the most fascinating perspective was not of the patient, but of the doctor. A panel of four medical oncologists all agreed that one single patient can have a powerful impact on their motivation and their love of a tough business. Listen to a paraphrased version of their panel discussion.

> Angry patients [stinkers] stomp into oncology exam rooms and chemo suites ranting, "Doctor, why must you put me through this agony? I am as sick as a dog. Just leave me alone." Most days, by 4:00 p.m. a cancer doctor is ready for early retirement but first, Mrs. Anderson waits patiently in Room #3. Doctor shuffles into her cubicle—beaten, worn. Patient greets Doctor with the warmest smile. Doctor and Patient start talking about grandchildren and the thrill of witnessing their achievements. Patient then gives a full account of scaring customers in the hair color aisle at the local drug store. Doctor describes the fiasco of his son's muffler falling off in rush hour traffic. Hearty belly laughs ring out from Room #3. Then, almost as an after-thought, Doctor and Patient discuss recent scan results, the progression of the disease, and what the next step might be. Patient is not surprised. Even so, laughter turns to quiet tears. Doctor holds Patient steady. Or is she holding Doctor steady? Dear, sweet Mrs. Anderson plants a kiss on *his* bald head, expressing thanks for his friendship. While she stands at the window making next week's appointment, the doctor promises himself to continue oncology practice for several more seasons.

Warning: please do not mistake me for dear, sweet Mrs. Anderson in Room #3. Even though I aim for a positive impact on my doctor, I can, on any given day, *lead* the stinker patients. My name is Connie Titus. Let me introduce Alan

S. Collin, M.D., my handsome, humorous medicine man (dance instructor).

To protect the identity and feelings of people involved, some names, locations, and, in a few places, minor details have been changed. However, these incidents are based on a true story and hopefully speak truth greater than any particulars surrounding them.

Now, step through the open clinic door and watch a Jewish man-doctor and his lopsided Gentile create fancy footsteps. Their attuned collaboration keeps the music playing for both.

Are you ready? Here we go, here we go!

Connie

Connie Thompson Titus

One hopeless night, about year six, I wrote this letter and tucked it in my last wish box. For some odd reason—don't ask why—it strikes me as a suitable beginning for this storybook.

Date: Uncertain

Dear Alan S. Collin, My Man-Doctor:

Here you have it, sir. Final communication, true confession, a speech after it's all over, my valedictorian address.

Why the term *final?* If you hold this letter in your hand, my husband, Neal, is dutifully distributing last greetings to important people. It is a good indication our work together is finalized. Have I avoided truth previously? Read on, with caution. What is over? Let me spell it out: *My life, as we know it, is over.* Who elected me valedictorian? I did. A woman with cancer can be whatever she wants. You probably agree my grade-point average ranked consistently high in your classroom. Consider me qualified.

Let us now review our doctor-patient, love-hate-love relationship, shall we?

Confession #1: Eventually you made an impression on me, but at first I did not want you nor like you. Your partner, Dr. Ivan Novelli, treated my daughter for a temporary blood condition. I knew him somewhat and asked my surgeon for a referral to him.

Friends urged us to seek a second opinion with a woman oncologist in Port Orange. Dr. Susan Mitchell, a breast cancer survivor herself, soothed our anxieties with her personal experience. She moved to first choice.

Neal and I had little say in this matter, though. Insurance companies rule with preferred provider lists and rejected Dr. Mitchell. My surgeon, Dr. Cappelletti, stomped his foot, insisting upon you. He mentioned communication track records and matching personality. So I was stuck with you and you were stuck with me in your musty, claustrophobic, badly-in-need-of-a-paint-job Ormond Beach office.

Would you like to hear my first assessment of Dr. Alan S. Collin?

Who is this man with dark circles under his eyes? He looks like he hasn't slept in a week. Is he healthy? And gosh, maybe someone should slip him the name of a good barber. Why does he spend my initial visit inquiring how medically informed I am? He cracks himself up with corny jokes. I don't understand them. I don't understand him. Hmm. Who is this man?

A couple of months later, probably in the face of danger, a tender moment presented itself. Dark circles, bad hair, and questionable jokes faded behind sensitivity. In the blink of a misty eye, I decided to want you and like you.

One morning appointment you found my frame twisted and bent—the result of wrestling with a heavy-weight slow cooker. Thank you for gentle care. Neal said it sounded as if you quoted pleasing jargon from my list of acceptable doctor behavior.

But during each office visit, whether you pleased me or made me madder than a hornet, I reaped the same benefits. Talking things over and having you touch me in familiar places (especially inside my head) stirred my soul's chemistry into a healing current. Healing currents transmit regeneration. Not a cure, mind you. I know, you know, and God knows you cannot cure cancer.

Our whole doctor-patient relationship was similar to touching the hem of Jesus' cloak. Oftentimes I received enough strength to pick up my bedroll and stroll another mile. On madder-than-hornet days there were no cloaks or tender touches, but the benefit of contact remained effective. These healing encounters set off positive sparks inside me. Perhaps my company triggered you into high gear, too.

I hope a comparison to Jesus does not insult a Jewish man-doctor. It is the highest compliment I can speak.

True confession #2: Some doctors get themselves confused with God, including you. Have a look.

Since we are connected by the sea, you Pisces you, I speak in a seafaring accent. Early on, my husband and I addressed you as captain of my ship. To date, you may still think you are captain of my ship. Sorry. You were demoted somewhere along the way. Or was it faulty casting on my part? The Captain of my ship is, was, and always has been God, the Great Physician. He appointed you chief navigator, Neal as first mate, and so on.

Now, characteristics of a chief navigator include grit and valor, vigor and amusement, and maybe even a New York shoulder shrug now and then. This is so you. In the course of your navigation, these components molded my sea legs.

And according to my church family, sturdy sea legs planted me securely on The Rock. People looked up to me spiritually. But none of them accompanied me behind closed doors on dark nights when I lost footage. Neither would they approve of whom I summoned for help.

Rather than cry out to the Lord, my Captain, I replayed the command in *your* voice. One simple recall seemed to calm the sea and nudge me ahead to my post. The trouble is that post was located on sinking sand, and my solace was short lived. Once I learned how to send desperate pleas God's way, replaying the command in *his* voice, a stance on solid rock came naturally. From there I could truly inspire.

King David writes about such salvation: "He lifted me out of the slimy pit, out of the mud and mire; he set my feet on a rock and gave me a firm place to stand" (Psalm 40:2, NIV). King David is talking about God, not any doctor. I hereby relieve you, Alan S. Collin, M.D., from the burden. Doctors do not need to assume the role of God, lifting folks up on rocks and such.

The true Ship Captain steered my vessel to your clinic's safe harbor. Referral to your watchful care was not a case of insurance ruling or Cappelletti getting his way (again). It was clearly God ruling and God getting his way (again). He organized you and me together on Nottingham Drive for good reason. I appreciate your accepting the assignment.

Confession of truth #3: I've got a crush on you, sweetie pie, Linda Ronstadt style.[1] I think it began that day you handed me a crazy prescription to dance. Remember? Despite my skepticism, flat-out refusals, and clumsy attempts, you really opened me up to so much more living. I learned that if the sun rises on a lady's fancy movement, a beautiful rhythm can set in for her day, and the next day, and a whole host of days, until she's blown all professional predictions out of the water.

It's only fitting that I ask you now: Alan S. Collin, M.D., may I have this celebrative dance? Come on, let's pretend. What? You don't hear any music? After all you taught me on this subject? Step closer and take my hand. Music resonates from my heart and soul, even now. Watch out, though. I like to lead. There may be dipping and spinning when you least expect it. Please wear argyle socks.

Fare thee well, my man-doctor. Remember me. I pray you've known all along how much I love you and thank God for you. My love and thanksgiving (and dancing) lives on, though you won't see me in the office on Tuesdays anymore.

May the Lord bless and keep you encouraged in your healing work.

Love,

Connie

Connie

P.S. Now you may ask why a mixed-up artist begins her story with the end. I'll tell you. Our God who designates appropriate seasons for everything under the sun also declares: "The end of a matter is better than its beginning…" (Ecclesiastes 7:8, NIV). That means I've come a long way, baby.

Thursday, February 6, 1997
Re: Connie B. Titus
D.O.B. 3/18/54
Referred by: Cappelletti

Alan S. Collin, M.D.:

I entered Stage Left suffering the sudden onset of a lethal disease and burial of a body part. How did our first office visit measure up?

Personally, I want to try again. With me in a post-diagnostic stupor and my husband, Neal, in his alarmed state of mind, we sat like a double bump on a log, too green to formulate intelligent questions about this thing called cancer.

You? Your main concern was my knowledge of medical terminology, being that I am employed by a general surgeon. You wanted to determine what you can and cannot slip by me, I suppose.

What did we talk about? Did we discuss surgical findings, statistics, or the particular strain of my disease? Have you investigated scan impressions and pathology results? If these factors did not make their way to our initial table, we should try again. Now I know why it is suggested patients tape oncology visits or come toting notebooks and sane secretaries.

When I am confused or in trouble, I do well to write it down—so get ready. If our working relationship continues for any length of time, you will need a big box for letters. I know. Competent, busy physicians don't have time to read personal letters from patients. Too bad. Behold your first installment.

The history notes below may assist you with other Inflammatory Breast Carcinoma (IBC) patients. Whoa. That brings up an excellent question. Do you have any other IBC patients? Long-time surgeon Dr. Cappelletti records only one other case and he won't tell me what happened to her.

Near Christmas I developed shooting pains in the left chest—heartburn due to rich holiday chocolate. Early January I rolled over onto a hardened, hot-to-the-touch, and swollen left breast. I was due for a yearly exam. If anyone asks, squishing a painful breast just about did me in. Mammography simply noted increased density. An ultrasound sent no red flags. Dr. Cappelletti and I agreed on breast infection, yet antibiotics and hot compresses did not relieve the symptoms. A week later his longest needle could not aspirate any fluid. We scheduled an incision and draining procedure at the hospital using local anesthetic.

General anesthesia was a last-minute change, and I am thankful. My surgeon cut into a big mess. I understand he stopped midstream to phone Dr. Morrison, my employer, and told him the situation did not look good.

On the recovery gurney with one blurry eye open, I asked Cappelletti if he found much fluid. He shook his head no. The disjointed conversation that followed did not concern me, and I told him so. "Cancer? Take my breast in three days? Take it where? There must be a mistake. You mixed me up with the lady in the next bed. I have no family history of breast cancer. Breast cancer is not painful—I suffered pain. The mammogram and ultrasound did not read suspicious for cancer. I am here with an infection. So you see, it is not me you are talking about. With all due respect, sir, check the chart again, please."

No mistake.

I will now rattle off the extent of my medical terminology: A modified radical mastectomy of the left breast was conducted January 27. Pathology reported Inflammatory Breast Carcinoma, a rare and aggressive strain making up only two to four percent of the entire breast cancer society. Margins were clean. Axillary lymph node dissection indicated thirteen of twenty nodes positive for malignancy. I am pre-menopausal and ER/PR negative. I agree. This does not look good. *Danger, Will Robinson!* [2]

Dr. Collin: Are you up for this challenge? Is Dr. Cappelletti still your friend? Am I your best research project thus far? Do you think I'll live, say, longer than six months, or do you even talk about such things? Why am I lost in space or stuck in such a melodrama? What did I do wrong? Are you healthy? Getting enough sleep? What are those dark circles about?

I have an urge to fasten my seatbelt, literally. Up to this point I've been breaking the law; I do not care to crash into a Floridian alligator-infested canal and not be able to get my seatbelt off. Secure strapping for the ride seems suddenly important now.

One of eight women will be called to the cancerous-breast boxing ring. They chose me from the lineup. I scurried through the house in search of a Bible I had not opened since Christmas 1976. Desperate times call for desperate measures. Last night I flipped through thin pages for an answer to "why me, why not the lady in the next bed?"

I was born and raised with a solid Christian upbringing, yet I am Bible illiterate, so it is pretty weird how the following verse caught my eye. "This will make possible the next step, which is for you to enjoy other people and to like them, and finally you will grow to love them deeply" (2 Peter 1:7, TLB). Is the underlying purpose of my melodrama to meet a new cast and crew? Well, cancer is giving me a chance to meet other people. I'm not sure how many I will enjoy.

This evening, ten days and seven hours later, I will survey for the first time the surgeon's work—my cut-up, naked body. I haven't been able to look at it. My husband viewed the new landscape. You checked it out Tuesday morning. It must not be too grotesque, or you guys would have run off screaming.

Thanks for being open to second opinions. I see Dr. Susan Mitchell in Port Orange Monday afternoon. But first, Cappelletti will install an infusaport in my chest tomorrow morning. We will meet again with you on Tuesday, February 11. Be prepared to answer the non-scientific questions above.

Wee, my fast-paced saga proceeds.

With weak and timid spirit,

Connie

Connie Beth Thompson Titus

P.S. If I may be so bold, even though I just claimed to be weak and timid: You...uh...need a haircut. Dave's Barber on Southwest Federation Highway is close to your office. You can drive there at lunchtime. [Smile]

Sunday, February 9, 1997
Re: Connie B. Titus
D.O.B. 3/18/54
Referred by: Cappelletti

Dr. Collin,

Your patient history form leaves little room for essentials. Before we talk about any treatment, please study my chemical makeup thus far.

I am dotted swiss and seersucker, black patent leather shoes, and fancy panties; I am forever plaid; I am saddle shoes, barrettes, and baby beers from the A&W Root Beer Stand.

I am a shiny blue Huffy bicycle capable of high speed, a metal lunch pail with milk money, a bomb scare, and a polio vaccine; I am a Brownie camera, a Brownie Girl Scout, and a chewy brownie (in my metal lunch pail).

I am Tiddly-Winks, Jacks, Hopscotch, Silly Putty, Paint by Number, and View Master; I am a jump rope with red handles that give way to rip out Cassie Walker's front teeth.

I am a Sunday school soloist singing "Jesus Loves Me" with all my heart, even though I have no idea who I am singing about.

I am related to Mr. Potato Head and Chatty Cathy, Captain Kangaroo, Dick, Jane, Spot, Sally, and Father Knows Best; I am a Barbie doll mixed with skullduggery in the closet; I am old Mr. and Mrs. Cotter's pesky visitor on their porch swing—he with his pipe, she with her knitting, me talking a mile a minute.

I am an acorn, an autumn leaf; I am a lilac, a tulip, and a peony; I am several litters of furry, purring kittens; I am a bonfire and fried potatoes on camp stoves; I am a tree house and a pink fort.

I am a black inner tube, a Coppertone tan, a beach ball,

and the card game Canasta; I am a spillway and forever a resident of a cottage on the waterfront.

I am a flutaphone, a licorice stick, brass, and sax; I am Gidget, The Monkees, and Ringo; I am a hip-huggin', short-skirted, wide-legged, tie-dyed, cloggin', and love-beaded flower child; I am a yellow chiffon prom dress wrapped in a borrowed white fur; I am white bucks and plumes, and I am a pair of flowered panties flying high on the flag pole at Band Camp Wakonda.

Most importantly, please make note, I am the blue garter girl. The band boys said so.

Now that you've got all that straight…birthright, birth order, and spirituality figure into my score.

Is a child of God allowed to consider astrology? March is my birth month. I simply cannot ignore the characteristics of the Piscean sign. They are too real.

An ideal day for a Pisces woman includes music, theater, film, photography, writing, and/or psychology. I am a woman of contradictions because the Piscean symbol is two fish swimming in opposite directions. I am fragile yet quite capable of fending for myself. Weak points include the lymphatic system, the feet, and super sensitivities to pollutants. My walking antenna picks up all the prevailing emotions of my surroundings, and I take the shape into which I am poured. Emergency relief comes from any body of moving water: a stream, waterfall, ocean, shower, or public fountain. Remember the beautiful blond in the public fountain scene of *Under the Tuscan Sun*?[3] Yeah, I want to be just like her, graceful and calm, with a good-looking guy to rescue me.

Even though I have three older sisters, I represent another generation, causing me to behave as an only child. I like to establish strong contact with the teacher. I wish to be in the limelight, under the guidance and protection of older people and people in positions of authority. Superiors, colleagues, and friends are to be what my parents were for me. Please, please, please make me your dearest child.

Whew. This is a big bill. Can you fill it? No, you cannot

fill it. If every only-child patient demanded this from you, you would be a dead man.

My spirituality can be summed up in the following paragraph. After Neal and I moved to Florida, an introduction to happy hour nearly ruined my sweet family life. Double doors of a local church stood wide open for folks like me, and I did go inside—alone. There I met up with beautiful parishioners, and to this day, we enjoy (what I consider) the most important facets of worship: hugging, harmonizing, and eating endless covered dishes. Last Sunday my name was listed in their bulletin under prayer concerns. These people are calling now, with a different tone, a certain degree of intensity. They talk about power, and grace, and faith. Why do I sense I'm standing on the edge of some kind of spiritual transformation? So I've got cancer. Let's get back to covered-dish luncheons.

I do feel better writing down the inner chemistry of Connie Titus. Digging deep to my roots builds a bit of security. Maybe there is a survivor in there after all.

The biggest problem is my red plaid dress. It now hangs crooked on the left side. What can you do about this?

Signed, a forever plaid patient,

Connie

Connie Titus

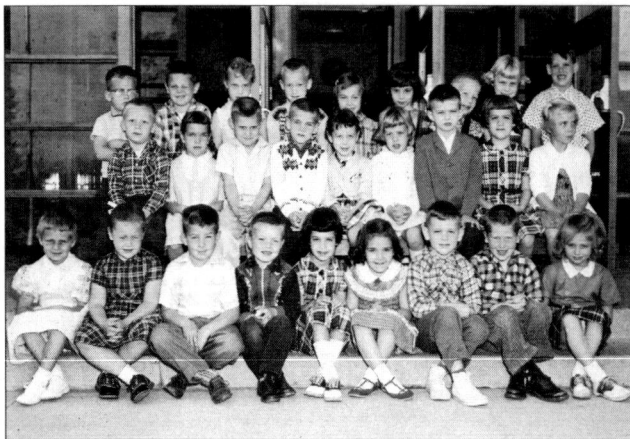

Mrs. Heffelfinger's (Plaid) Kindergarten Class, Northeastern Elementary, Bellefontaine, Ohio, 1959. "O Lord, you alone are my hope; I've trusted you from childhood" (Psalm 71:5, TLB).

Courtesy of Bellefontaine City School Photographer

Monday, February 10, 1997
Re: Connie B. Titus
D.O.B. 3/18/54
Referred by: Cappelletti

Dear Dr. C:

Our visit with Dr. Susan Mitchell today got me thinking. Do you know she is a breast cancer survivor? What happens when oncologists face cancer on the home front: spouse, parent, child, self? I shudder at the thought. You've chosen to share in daily sufferings of decent people, and your eyes show sadness. I imagine any personal cancer diagnosis would prompt you to jump off the edge of the earth. Why wait for staging, prognoses, or treatment options?

But if you wrestled with this beast in your own backyard, sensitivities toward patients and caregivers should heighten—big time. We would win from your adversity.

Dr. Collin, I'm just learning how to pray. I ask God to protect you and yours from cancer.

Be compassionate now, with a man grieving over his wife's breast.

Our commotion started January 24, a rainy Friday morning. Neal sat alone in the surgical waiting room. He did not feel it necessary to bring a stable friend, not for a simple infection. Dr. Cappelletti was to drain my abscess. Recovery would see that I peed and dressed, in that order. Neal could then drive me home, tuck me in, and get on back to work. That was the plan.

But why did the plan take so long?

Cappelletti finally approached my husband, dragging a lead balloon. No fanfare.

"Your wife has cancer."

Oh, the size of the knife that cut through Neal's chest

wall. The messenger turned and walked away. No one braced my husband or picked up his bloody pieces.

I opted to spend the night in the hospital. An inflamed biopsy left me with a drain sticking out of my side. Neal went home to cry his eyes out. That evening he brought the children to look at me with their big, wet eyes. No one said much. Dr. Cappelletti appeared long enough to explain Monday's mastectomy, prognosis dependent on lymph node involvement and scheduling of comprehensive scans. I signed a consent form for amputation. Again, no one said much. The sky turned mega dark. My family gathered their science-fiction information, backed up in slow motion, and filed down the hallway. Neal cried his eyes out some more. I tried to cry too. Nothing came out.

The next morning reality shot through me like a bazooka. Tears flowed freely. I stood at the hospital window, waiting, watching for my lover man. "Dear God, I hope he doesn't forget. Today is a great walking away place for him. Some men do, you know?"

Looking out that institutional window, I wondered why or how people were still driving, still walking about. Birds fluttered in and around the clouds, probably singing. The sun rose in plain sight. Humanity and nature apparently have no respect for sorrow. On his way into town, Neal sensed the world spinning as usual and shook his head with dismay. After twenty-three years of marriage, it is proper for man and wife to think alike.

He made it. My lover man. He was ashen-faced, but stood tall beside me, carefully guiding me and that nasty, blood-filled drain into a buttoned-down blouse and a pair of jeans that wouldn't quite come together over a bloated tummy. I wondered, *Will he still think me pretty?*

We headed home in the Dodge truck. What a bumpy ride. A post-surgical patient sporting a drain longs for a vehicle with a set of good shocks, but I kept my mouth shut. Neither one of us whistled or smiled like we normally do in the Dodge truck. We were clumsy with each other, trying to digest the idea of more surgery in forty-eight hours.

Oh, the dreaded drain. How funny, although the pain wasn't funny. The surgeon released me with a flimsy bandage, so every time I moved about or took a deep breath, the drain shifted between angry tissues. Ouch. I did not want to look at it, much less empty the thing. Neal had been through the mill and back; I could not ask him to handle such a gross tool. I called every nurse friend between Florida and Ohio. No nurse in her right mind stays home on a Saturday night, so we were alone with this thing.

My precious husband figured out the mechanics; he drained it and tightened the bandage, which relieved the pain. I awarded him the honorable title of Drain Master. Overnight, Neal O. Titus transformed into an efficient nursemaid and coach. Thus began the first intimate chapter of a different volume of matrimony.

Gosh, I married the nicest guy. I think God teamed me up with him. We will face together, whatever. When there is stumbling involved, two are always better than one, picking up the pieces, warming, conquering.

Dr. Collin, after our second opinion consult, we choose you to join our team. We shall make it a three-legged race. Along that train of thought, can I quote a beautiful wise (short) story out of my Living Bible? It is interesting to read relevant ideas written thousands of years ago.

> Two can accomplish more than twice as much as one, for the results can be much better. If one falls, the other pulls him up; but if a man falls when he is alone, he's in trouble. Also, on a cold night, two under the same blanket gain warmth from each other, but how can one be warm alone? And one standing alone can be attacked and defeated, but two can stand back-to-back and conquer; three is even better, for a triple-braided cord is not easily broken.
>
> Ecclesiastes 4:9-12 (TLB)

Yes, let us be a triple-braided cord. Please and thank you.

Praying is downright awkward for me, but may I say or write another prayer for you? "Blessed art thou, O Lord our God, King of the Universe, please protect Dr. Collin and his family from cancer, and please shield this good doctor from ever grieving over his wife's breast. Amen."

See you tomorrow,

Connie

Connie, the Drain Master's Wife

P.S. I am officially worried. Who is this person quoting scripture and writing prayers? I used to be the one who smiled and quietly backed away from conversations about God. Is this a side effect of cancer?

Wednesday, February 12, 1997
Re: Connie B. Titus
D.O.B. 3/18/54
Referred by: Cappelletti

Alan S. Collin, M.D., P.A.,

You've got mail.

I know what M.D. and P.A. stand for, but how about the S? What middle name did your Mom and Daddy give you? Are your parents alive and well? Do you see them/talk to them often? How have they influenced your life's work? Are you sick and tired of my questions?

Sorry, but not really. If you and I engage in a working relationship, I should know who you are. And while I heal, seek second opinions, prepare for the trek, I will spill my guts out in plain view for you. Is this all right?

Today is my Father's birthday. "Happy Birthday, Daddy." His body lies next to Mom in the cold, hard ground of Ohio, yet my religious training says their spirits dance together somewhere warm and glorious. Sadly for me, there is no phone number listed for somewhere warm and glorious. And they forgot to leave a forwarding address.

A rocky road stretches far up ahead. How do I proceed without parents? They have been dead so long I should be used to it. Older sisters try to assume the parental roles, but only Moms and Daddies can fix desperation. My good parents had a flair for gentle understanding and guidance, sprinkled with high praise. I really need them. Will someone please slip me Mom and Daddy's new long-distance phone number?

Since my folks left town, may I cry the mastectomy blues with you? Remember, an only child requires authority figures to act like parents. Dr. Cappelletti doesn't want to hear it. Yes, surgery was two weeks ago, and you can rightly raise your voice: "Get over it already!" I will write my pain down on paper anyway. You can take it or leave it.

Cappelletti downgraded me to one breast. He set out to remove my left breast, but I think he broke every rib in the process. I am in agony. Also, when I move about, I swear there is a needle sticking in the back of my left arm. I have asked Neal and the nurses to look for it.

Oh boy, two drains. My beloved Drain Master kicks into double duty.

Demerol puts a smile on my face but slows my breathing and blood pressure down to about nothing. Connie Titus warns against swallowing narcotics on an empty stomach.

Procedures following a word like cancer include scans of the head, neck, chest, abdomen, pelvis, bones, and every particle in between. Gee whiz. With all the radioactive, nuclear injections, God shall have no trouble finding me in the dark.

Reach to Recovery representatives want me to exercise, but it hurts. Besides, who will want me to reach a bowl on the top shelf if I am full of cancer? Let's wait for scan results.

A pink lady wheeled me by the hospital discharge office where they hand out payment plans like souvenirs. Great. I must pay money for this misery.

Family, friends, coworkers, and the community stand beside me and pray. They say God hears and delivers people from fear. I am so timid about talking with the Lord myself. I know not what or how to pray. If Mom and Daddy were alive, they'd instruct me on what the Good Book says on this subject: "In the same way, the Spirit helps us in our weakness. We do not know what we ought to pray for, but the Spirit himself intercedes for us with groans that words cannot express" (Romans 8:26, NIV).

B.C. (before cancer), in the throes of depression, I thought my family might be better off without me. Now I change my mind. Prospects of graduations, weddings, and grandchildren invite me to choose life. "Are you listening, God? Please, I fearfully and awkwardly hand this whole mess to you. I understand you are near to those who call upon you. Here I stand. Lord, could you see to it that Mom and Daddy know of my little problem? They must be with you in Ohio's heaven. Look them up, please, Alinette and Lewis. Thanks. Oh, and watch over my husband and children who are frightened way worse than me. I will be forever grateful."

Dr. Collin, call your Mom or Daddy today; no one knows what tomorrow brings. Earth, Wind & Fire gives good advice in their song "Celebrate": "Celebrate what you're thinking of, time ain't long, soon we'll be moving on, moving on."[4]

Thanks for listening,

Connie

Connie

Sunday, March 9, 1997
Re: Connie B. Titus
D.O.B. 3/18/54
Referred by: Cappelletti

Hello Doc,

Before our last office visit, I did some homework. You probably hate to hear this from patients. It cuts into your degree of manipulation.

I designed for myself a nice little treatment package. You should thank me for streamlining your job. I will undergo a conventional chemotherapy regimen combined with prayer, diet, and visualization—right here in my hometown. Sounds like a winner, huh?

Wrong.

"This is serious," you say. "We have to take an aggressive approach. I want you to consider Stem Cell Rescue (SCR) at Duchess University in Alabama. I can set up a consultation next week."

You spent considerable time supporting this recommendation and sent us home with a scary booklet. Neal and I agreed to visit an institution that implements the transplant procedure but one closer to home. Thursday we met with Dr. Jacob Robertson at St. Luke Regional in Daytona Beach.

Between the booklet and our visit with Dr. Robertson, there is no way to paint a pretty picture of SCR's jazz.

Correct me if I'm wrong. The patient spends about two months in or around the facility. Stem Cell Rescue is coupled with high-dose chemotherapy leaving the patient a toxic bag of bones with numerous intensified complications—fatal complications in some cases. If the complications don't kill you, they are treated with, oh my gracious, more drugs.

After discharge, the assessment for organ damage begins. For instance, the lung is often affected and treated with four to six weeks of cortisone, which brings its own set of undesirable side-effects. SCR seems like one big, frightful option. No one walks away normal.

And SCR is still fairly new as far as breast cancer is concerned. There are no studies assuring long-term benefits.

In my opinion, SCR disrupts household routine and financial security, causing more stress, causing more cancer. I would need to leave my job that provides family health insurance coverage. Neal, as caregiver, would have to take an indefinite leave-of-absence from the paint store. There would be no alternative but to place our young son in the care of a friend because no family members reside in Florida.

Neal was impressed with Dr. Robertson and staff. And of course the husband wants his wife to pursue any and all avenues to stay alive. His vote is *yes*.

Let's see, should I:

1. Go with conventional therapy, risking inevitable, but not necessarily imminent, death from the disease?

   or

2. Agree to Stem Cell Rescue, which offers a reasonable chance of cure via a painful and frightening procedure that may be fatal?

What fun is this? "Dear Lord, send us wisdom pronto. Your Holy Word promises wisdom."

> For the Lord grants wisdom! His every word is a treasure of knowledge and understanding. He grants good sense to the godly—his saints. He is their shield, protecting them and guarding their pathway. He shows how to distinguish right from wrong, how to find the right decision every time.
>
> Proverbs 2:6-9 (TLB)

Hmm. God "grants good sense to the godly—his saints." That leaves me out.

Stem Cell Rescue rubbed me the wrong way from the

start, but after our trip to Daytona Beach and Neal's voiced support, it became a consideration. Boy, do I get grumpy in dark corners with sharp angles. I shot a desperate cry to God.

On the morning of my Mom's birthday, March 7, I believe the Lord unveiled a clear picture. I am a traditional, old-fashioned girl who is most comfortable with moderation. Do not take me away from my children, my home, or my support system. If I need hospitalization, it should be here, where I have developed a large circle of friends. Quality living, or some semblance thereof, is half my healing. A ball game, Sunday fellowship, or a few hours in the office…this is who I am. If recurrence knocks in the future, we will deal with it then.

Convincing Neal of God's clear picture was slightly rough, but he will come to like the idea very soon.

My vote on SCR is *no, thank you*. Please sir, set me up with a cocktail in your claustrophobic office. I will report for the Multiple Gated Acquisition scan (MUGA scan) tomorrow and see you Tuesday.

Is a MUGA scan like a mug shot, a front and side view of each of your inmates?

Sincerely,

Connie

Connie, a traditional, conventional, moderate patient (so far)

Tuesday, March 25, 1997
Re: Connie B. Titus
D.O.B. 3/18/54
Referred by: Cappelletti

Dr. Collin, Sir:

The MUGA scan showed my heart good and strong. Therefore, you set us on a launch pad cleared for take-off on Tuesday, March 11, 1997.

That morning Nurse Nicole ushered Neal and me to your small chemotherapy room under construction. Or was it the gas chamber? Anyway, a large bag of red fluid hung on a silver pole with my name on it. Oh, boy.

Nicole introduced us to Sadie, another first-timer. Sadie's silver pole also held a big red bag, thus her anxious expression. Nicole warned us not to share horror stories. But all nervous women must chatter, so we did.

"Oh, my gosh!"

"You are kidding!"

Listen to our similarities: Sadie and I were diagnosed with breast cancer on the same side, days apart; our birthdays are the same day, ten years apart; both families moved to Florida in 1979; Sadie and her husband, Jeff, enjoy country wood crafting; in fact, Jeff nervously flipped through their favorite pattern catalog, which happens to be *our* favorite pattern catalog. Our husbands look alike with gray beards, receding hairlines, glasses. They sat next to each other with similar gentle dispositions, having no earthly idea what was ahead for them.

Is Sadie a soul mate? Are we carbon copies of one another for a reason? Very interesting timing, don't you think? Do you believe in signs, Dr. Collin? That, to me, was a bold sign that I am where I am supposed to be. God might even be in control.

Sadie and I tolerated your big red bag of fluid relatively well. And of course our conversation was a comfortable distraction.

If you record side effects (please do!), the first week a few waves of nausea, weakness, and unidentifiable sensations came over me, but my household never missed a beat. On day eight, however, I was one sick puppy. Nausea, vomiting, diarrhea, severe headache, chills, mouth sores—every possibility printed in the chemo pamphlet attacked me. I felt bad enough to phone your office. Nurse Nicole explained my symptoms indicated dropping white counts. Sure enough, on day twelve my white blood count registered 2.2. Here we go. "Beware of infection," Nicole cautioned. Breathing became a labored effort and possibly a lethal function.

Did I really agree to this? Did I accept your invitation to a cocktail party every twenty-one days for the next six months?

You cleared us for take-off, all right. Right now I want to take off in any other direction. I should take off from the bedroom to the study. I understand successful chemo patients educate themselves.

Later,

Connie

Connie B. Titus

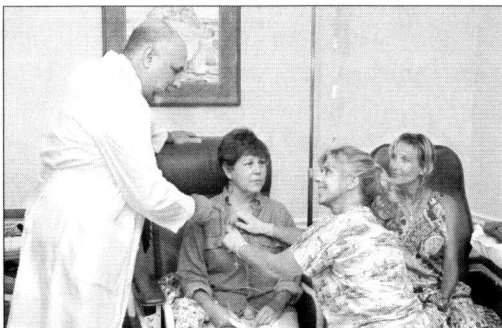

Dr. Collin, Nurse Nicole, Patient Connie, and new friend Sadie assemble for first chemotherapy cocktail party.

Courtesy of Photographer Jerry Brewer

Friday, April 4, 1997
Re: Connie B. Titus
D.O.B. 3/18/54
Referred by: Cappelletti

Dear Doctor:

Thanks for poking and prodding and sticking me with needles on Tuesday. Were you only poking fun? Tuesday was April Fool's Day.

Do oncologists allow emotional talk or should I see a shrink? The idea of family counseling appeals to me, but I would have to drag Neal kicking and screaming. What I record below might be normal lopsided jitters, and you may have a quick fix. If so, please fix us all. If not, write a referral. You can file this letter or toss it, whatever floats your boat.

Tension runs rampant at 151 Windemere Drive. My husband will be the first to crack. He jokes about reserving a rubber room in our local insane asylum. I fail to appreciate that type of humor. Yet I realize that his sleepless nights, multi-tasking days, and absolutely no love-making encounters marked on the calendar might drive him there for real.

Neal told me this morning he has not slept since January 24. Nightmares of cancerous lead balloons make him thrash in the bed.

He drives to town for daytime work and drives to the country for nighttime work, with no recollection of either one. Laundry, meal preparation, assorted housework, and mommy chores are now Neal's responsibilities because I lie around like a slug. And he makes all decisions for I have no opinion. Despite operational overload, he somehow dries tears, plumps pillows, and runs to the corner store for ginger ale and Jell-o, getting very little affection in return. A sad life for him.

Caryn, our twenty-year-old daughter, stays out late, sleeps

late, works long hours, and keeps a friend in tow at all times. She is, therefore, protected from me and my disease. Granted, everyone deserves a defense mechanism. When encouraged by family or friends to take good care of Mom, my little girl responds, "I have no choice!" Ouch. That hurts.

We are open with our son, Ron. He is still very young and doesn't seem to ask questions. It is hard to tell what goes through his eleven-year-old mind. Sometimes he reveals his stress with inappropriate behavior.

Me? I behave inappropriately also. What I think and say and do annoys people. I am no longer Connie Titus but a physical, emotional, and financial drain. As a cancer patient, I deem myself unemployable, uninsurable, and un-enjoyable for the rest of my life.

My job with Dr. Morrison creates dilemma. Physically, I am not able to work more than twenty hours a week, but they pay me full-time salary. Reaping what I do not sow brings guilt.

Aggravation is at its worst behind the wheel. City and county motorists should scatter between here and there for I have no patience. Neal offered to install a railroad tie onto the front of my Grand Marquis, which would allow me to push aside all those who don't know where they're going. *Get out of my way!* Everybody, everywhere, must get out of my way.

I worked hard preparing myself and my family for the physical jolt of disease and treatment, never giving emotions much thought. It should have been the other way around. Spiritually, I am in a comfortable lot, yet depression finds a way in. Not only do I (we) struggle with disease, chemical effects, and unknown outcome, but dreaded menopause is on its way. Doesn't menopause drive women crazy all by itself? And Florida's heat is a nice touch. I have been hot-blooded since childhood.

Can I do it? Will my family survive? Mom usually glues the family together during crisis. What happens if Mom *is* the crisis? Preachers versed in the Good Book say all things are possible with God. Do you agree, Dr. Collin?

Any helpful hints are appreciated, or you may set me up with a shrink of your choice.

Regards from your emotional, high-strung patient #25561,

Connie

Mrs. Connie Titus

Thursday, April 24, 1997

Doc:

Your expertise is the drug plan, but certainly you must lend a sympathetic ear on the subject of self-image. Can you sit through a graphic letter without developing a nervous twitch? Notice how I choose to write rather than discuss it face to face. That way I don't have to witness your nervousness or stop before I am finished.

From here on I drop reference notes in the upper left-hand corner of my letters. You know who I am, my birth date, and the scoundrel who handed me over. Actually, anonymity would be good today.

A breast is not important. I tell God I would rather lose a breast than my eyesight, hearing, or a limb. But truly, my human heart grieves for the suppleness the surgeon carved and tossed aside. I suppose it sits on a shelf in a lab. My right breast is lonely. My right breast is at risk. I frantically check it daily.

I should say, "It matters not, I have another one." But the blatant truth is that it does matter. God made two, I want two. Neal reminds me I have two breasts. One may sit in a drawer all night, but I own two breasts. All of a sudden I am obsessed with beauty, glamour, and sex appeal, of which I have none. No combination of jewelry, makeup, perfume, silk, or lace is going to fix this. How many one-breasted mannequins do you see donning flattering fashions? None. The lingerie shop is the worst. I could easily throw myself onto their floor in a weeping heap. We live in a two-breasted society, and I will never again fit in.

Oh, we like the prosthesis all right. It warms up to body temperature, presents a life-like bounce, looks symmetrical, and fits good in Neal's hand. But sometimes it will not stay in place. Little pockets must be sewn into bras and bathing suits. I like a good laugh too, but explaining what fell out of my top with a plop or what floats toward the diving board is something I would rather avoid.

Discomfort of a mastectomy and lymph node removal causes me to carry my left arm like Napoleon. Then Cappelletti installed an infusaport in the right chest wall, sinking it in deep for cosmetic reasons, causing me to carry the right arm like Napoleon as well. Neal constantly reminds me to put my arms down. This Napoleon stance appears rather conspicuous in the supermarket. Shoppers whisper, "What is her problem?" Ooh, I want to snap back, "I worked hard to get this way. Now, mind your own business!"

A Reach to Recovery representative said that unless I climb the walls (exercise), I will lose use of both arms. Pain prevented me from doing this at first. Then I wanted to wait for test results. If I were full of cancer, flexibility sure wouldn't matter. Scan results are lovely, though, so flexibility *does* matter and I climb the walls.

When lymph nodes are removed, any scratch, cut, bruise, bug bite, or sunburn becomes an infectious risk. Should I order one of those protective bubbles?

I told God another white lie. I said it wouldn't bother me to lose my hair. Wigs, hats, and headgear might be fun. I ordered a brunette wig. Before it came I spied a lady in your waiting room with the same color and style as what I ordered. She sat there like a zombie. United Parcel Service delivered my wig. I tried it on and saw, in my mirror, the zombie. That was the night before my forty-third birthday. I sobbed profusely. Neal paced outside the bedroom door, wringing his hands over my pathetic prayer. "Dear Lord, I made a mistake. My breast, my hair, I need them back, please, right this minute! Oh, God, I should be in the prime of my life, like my mom. Remember? She gave birth to me at age forty-three. But here I am, age forty-three, falling apart—one cell, one hair follicle at a time."

Oh, no. Can you believe it? I was shouting at God. Dr. Collin, I told you—I'm new at this prayer business.

Let me expand on hair loss. The brush is full with every stroke. I leave a trail behind me. On Easter Sunday I shampooed ever so gently, leaving me enough hair to style and spray heavily. Immediately after the worship service a whole handful fell out. I laughed and tried to give away remnants. Church buddies screeched and scattered. When home alone it was no laughing matter to me either. My femininity, my dignity, all my attractiveness goes down our shower drain. Hair sticks to a wet body, wet scars. I had no idea hair loss could be so traumatic. Am I vain?

Neal kept offering to put a shine on that thing (my head). At 8:00 p.m. last evening, with cold beer in hand (am I allowed to drink beer? Uh oh. Too late!), my husband pulled out his buzz saw and put a shine on that thing. Neal humors me, but my guess is this project hurt him more than me. We let the kids see me right away. Thank God for children. They cheered, "Mom is cool!" Dave Dravecky claims bald chemo heads scare unwanted door-to-door salesmen. I will give this a try.

You say Adriamycin, or *The Big Red One* as Neal refers to it, will throw a pre-menopausal woman into menopause after the first treatment, yet I had a period last week. You clarify. The ovaries start talking to each other after the first treatment. They decide exactly when to retire. Today I overheard my ovaries Orville and Ozzie hollering back and forth about retirement and/or uselessness. One is reluctant, as is my soul. This will end an era at too early an age. I am not sure I can handle menopausal hot flashes, crazy thoughts, and palpitations on top of chemo hot flashes, crazy thoughts, and palpitations, especially during the hot, buggy Florida summer. What have I got myself into?

On the subject of weight gain—ugghh. Cappelletti suggested I beef up for your treatments. Church ladies deliver four-course meals and I have an appetite. A bald head and round bottom reminds me of a bowling pin. Say what? I can walk briskly? Okay. When might I feel inspired to do this?

Sleeping is a struggle because the mind is a terrible thing. I agree with a comedian whose name escapes me. He said, "The mind should be stamped out in our lifetime!" Other sleepless reasons include twitches, aches, burning, and restless leg syndrome. Sometimes, though, I lay awake all night singing praises because I lived through another day.

So who is this woman?

I am torn but patched into a great specimen with a cute, man-made replacement part. I am wired for sound, or at least IV drips. I can grab a beer mug on the top shelf. I'm bald as a billiard ball, but it *is* great fun scaring salesmen. I contemplate the passage into middle age and grump around from interrupted sleep. But do not be sad for me. I get up, apply lipstick, and go to work every day at least for a couple hours. If I feel bad, I take a pill. I rest. I smile and laugh a lot. Praise God I am home for these treatments. I give him thanks for the small pleasures of fresh air, good appetite, hot showers, friendly check-up calls, back rubs, and the sound of my children bickering…and you, Doctor, a white knight in my corner. Yep, much goodness comes to me still.

I think the Potter is reworking me into another vessel as seems good to him; probably the best part, for the Potter, is my acknowledgement of his involvement, his interest (Inspired by Jeremiah 18:4, NIV).

How ya doin' with the nervous twitch?

From a torn, patched specimen,

Connie

Connie

Tuesday, April 29, 1997

Hey,

Connie Titus here—#25561 spinning out of control.

Chemo No. 3 was no picnic. You are right. Side effects accumulate and step up a notch. I lay awake too nauseated to sleep. Like a woman in labor, I focused on framed memories on the bedroom wall: my childhood home, the Hammond Theater, and Band Camp Wakonda (where my panties may still be flying on the flagpole). How did the young, healthy me get so sick?

Last week's treatment took me down and out sideways for about five days. Even the anti-nausea pills didn't help. When I am nauseated I could just die. I would rather push an eight-pound, ten-ounce freight train through the keyhole. During nausea and vomiting I stop regarding your chemo as helpful treatment and label it poison. This poison destroys every bit of good health that God put into me.

My white count dropped dangerously low this time around. You ordered shots of Neupogen to stimulate those dangerously low white cells, a shot each day for three days. All drugs have side effects. Neupogen affects only 23% with severe bone pain. Why, oh why, can't I be in the other 77%? Neupogen causes me horrid bone pain. If I turn or twist a certain way, my skeleton will splinter. Neal is not capable of cleaning up the mess. I will not ask him to. Do you have a skeleton repair team on call?

I will only take two shots, sir. Give my third shot to some needy person with my compliments.

Won't someone please write a song for me, a song that will stop the spinning? Bring in Earth, Wind & Fire singing "I'll Write a Song for You." "We're in a spinning top, where, tell me, will it stop, and what am I to say…there in your silent night, joy of a song's delight, I write a song for you."[5]

Signed,

Connie

Connie (Ms. Bone Pain, spinning out of control, waiting for a song)

Sunday, May 25, 1997

Dear Dr. Collin:

While you were out…what the heck is this?

During the last week of March, we noticed a bright red patch around the incision area. Each office visit since, you and I tried to determine if it was an allergic reaction to the prosthesis, a rash, or a reaction to the Adriamycin. The worst scenario would be Inflammatory Breast Carcinoma (IBC) coming back to haunt me. [Sigh] Actually, this is probably a good place to let out at least one cuss word, but I don't know you well enough.

Tuesday, May 6, you gave me a prescription cream and told me to forego the prosthesis; if it wasn't better in a week, I was to see Dr. Cappelletti or a dermatologist. Poof, you were gone for a two-week vacation. I fought a strong urge to grab hold of your pant leg and beg you to stay.

Maybe my imagination ran wild, but the redness appeared to be spreading even with the cream. I did not wait a full week to see Cappelletti. He grit his teeth.

My fear was his fear, and probably your fear too. Skin metastasis. He and I discussed "what if." One option was for him to excise the whole area, a 6 x 3 ½-inch patch, and do a skin graft. His other idea was radiation to the chest wall. Wish you were here! White counts were in range, so Dr. Cappelletti performed a biopsy on May 21. Sure enough, pathology proved another malignancy. He warned me twice that chemotherapy may not alter my condition. If this is Inflammatory Breast Carcinoma recurring after three courses of strong chemicals, what's next?

I think you'll agree hometown physicians know little about IBC. Therefore, if it pleases you, Dr. Collin, will you refer me to a specialist before any more treatments? A larger cancer center might see more of this rarity. Thank you.

Folks pray for me continually. People who seem to have a direct line say I will be fine. I want to be fine. I want to live long as a parent, a grandparent. I could even promise God to serve long as a faithful follower. Well, why don't I prove my faith right now by repeating to myself that I will be fine and dandy?

But God knows the Girl Scout in me strives to be prepared, so I prepare. Orchestration of my passing is underway. And when it is typed up nice and pretty, I can just as well tuck it in the last wish box, bottom left-hand desk drawer, for another thirty years.

Now you know what I have been doing the last two weeks—undergoing the knife and preparing to die.

Oh, forgive me. How was your vacation?

Still me,

Connie

Connie B. Titus
D.O.B. 3/18/54
Referred by: Cappelletti

Tuesday, May 27, 1997

Good Evening, Doctor Collin:

Our daughter's long-time best friend, Hettie, is a dear member of the Titus Family. She is predictable after all these years. When we gather for suspenseful movie night, within twenty minutes, Hettie squirms in her seat, removes herself for a drink, returns in the middle of a particularly tense scene, asking the same question, "How does this turn out?"

Even if we knew the outcome, we would not spoil it for her or anyone else in the room. Neal's pat answer is, "I don't know, Hettie. You should watch quietly and find out."

It is suspenseful movie night here on Windemere Drive. My cancer grows despite strong artillery. I am in the middle of a particularly tense scene, squirming in my seat. In an anxious, irritated tone I want to question somebody, anybody, "How does this turn out?" The suspense is killing me. Literally. My Father on his throne wants me to watch quietly and find out.

Thanks for meeting with us this morning. What a worried look on your face, though. And then the worried look transferred to our faces when you handed me that prescription to dance at daybreak. Neal said my forehead formed a question mark. Good night nurse, Dr. Collin! Have you lost your ever-lovin' mind? I can't dance. I can't even shuffle to the kitchen to pour myself a glass of milk. You want me to get up out of the bed when the sun comes up and do what?

You stood before us in your starched-white coat talking nonsense. "Connie, you come to me for advice. I want you to show the debilitating disease and treatment you are boss. Seek some enjoyment due you; lace up your dancing shoes. White cells will surely multiply in the process."

This is about as silly as prescribing cherry pie for migraines, coconut macaroons for diarrhea, or a bar of soap under the bed sheet for restless leg syndrome. Wait a minute, these ridiculous cures work for me.

I admit you are the one with an education. Your ways are probably higher than our ways. I asked you to tell us more.

"Stop seeking new landscape and get a new pair of eyes," you say.

"So it's more of a state of mind thing?"

"Yes." You instruct that if I am not physically able to jump out of bed and do a cha-cha on the porch, I should tell Neal to put in a jazzy CD and go through the motions in my head.

Well, these legs cannot support me right now, but I guess I can lie here and dream. My mom practiced dynamic imaging in her bed-ridden days.

You explained two important factors of successful patients. First, I must hear the music, meaning I must open my ears, eyes, and mind to life's possibilities. Second, I need to decide for myself how best to keep the music playing, which will strengthen my pulse and motivate. You stress that motivation is a personal matter. The neighbor's plan will not work for me.

How about this for starters? I'll imagine myself with a full head of hair, a whole and healthy body on stage with Earth, Wind & Fire.

"Now you're catchin' on!"

With this prescription to dance at daybreak, you want a groove to set in my shoes and light my fuse. In your practice, you've noticed when folks start to focus their minds on a healthy image, their bodies respond. And cancer patients need goals. Rugged times can be appealing if you have a goal.

You were on a roll this morning and offered a second prescription. "Don't ask why, ask how, or what is next." I read this same theory in *Breast Cancer? Breast Health! The Wise Woman Way*. "The Wise Woman asks 'How?' She knows that 'Why' leads to (and springs from) the erroneous belief that we can control our lives. 'How' helps us remember that we can participate fully in our lives no matter how out of control they seem. 'Why' points the finger of blame. 'How' points to the places we need to nourish."[6] Next time I come in with a long list of questions, I will not start them with *why*.

Back to dancing: Are you prepared to stand front and center in the chemo room and give an example? Yeah, buddy, get to it. I'll put Earth, Wind & Fire's "Let's Groove" on the phonograph and you can show us what you're made of.

> [Excerpt lyrics] Let this groove set in your shoes. Stand up, all right…let you know, girl, you're looking good, you are out of sight and all right. Move yourself and glide like a 747. Lose yourself in the sky among the clouds in the heavens. Stand up, all right. You will find peace of mind on the floor…share the spice of life. Let this groove set in your shoes. Stand up, all right.[7]

What a productive office visit. I am to dance at daybreak and ask how, not why. I think I can, I think I can, I think I can. Thanks for these prescriptions. And thanks for setting up a consultation appointment with Dr. Vince Channon. We see him Thursday.

"Lace up my dancing shoes, dear Lord of the Dance, and grant me the strength. Amen."

Have a good evening,

Connie

Connie

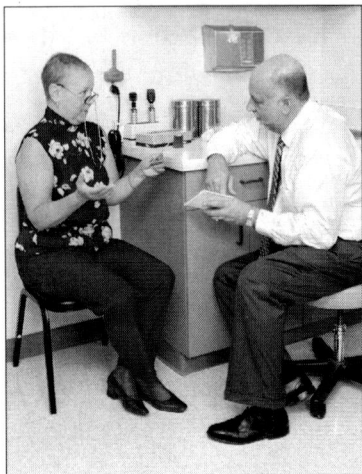

Dr. Collin hands over an unorthodox prescription for Patient Connie to dance first thing in the morning. Gazing over the top of her glasses with disbelief, Patient is not so patient—she wants to choke him with his necktie.

Courtesy of Photographer
Jerry Brewer

P.S. I don't understand what God is up to. His thoughts and ways are confusing, like yours. Why doesn't he slip someone a note, like Hettie? *How does this turn out, Hettie?* I do take solace knowing Biblical authors suffered the same confusion.

> For my thoughts are not your thoughts, neither are your ways my ways, declares the Lord. As the heavens are higher than the earth, so are my ways higher than your ways and my thoughts than your thoughts.
>
> Isaiah 55:8-9 (NIV)

> …no one knows the thoughts of God except the Spirit of God.
>
> 1 Corinthians 2:11 (NIV)

> As you do not know the path of the wind, or how the body is formed in a mother's womb, so you cannot understand the work of God, the Maker of all things.
>
> Ecclesiastes 11:5 (NIV)

Sunday, June 1, 1997

To My Knight in Starched-White Coating:

Professionals who admit they do not know all the answers earn my respect. I place another star in your signature for simply saying "I don't know." And heroism takes shape when you welcome second and third opinions. Thank you. Stay the way you are. I swayed to Earth, Wind & Fire's beat this morning, thinking of you. "Be ever wonderful, stay as you are…don't let the world change your mind."[8]

Thursday, we consulted with world-renowned breast cancer expert and your buddy, Dr. Vince Channon. Neal and I chuckle. He reminds us of that goofy guy on the sitcom *Mad About You*.[9] Dr. Channon will forward office notes; meanwhile you hold this layman's synopsis.

I came away bawling. And the man felt bad about it; he called me early the next morning at work to go over prospects of hope, something he said he had failed to do in the office. Duh. Tears gushed as he talked over my head suggesting treatment drugs foreign to me. Worse than that, this man lacked compassion. Neal and I viewed him as a scientist or a mathematician calculating cells and genes.

I suppose we did not give him a chance. You have spoiled us rotten with your bedside manner. And I shuffled in, as any newly-diagnosed victim suffering a rapid recurrence, wearing emotions on the tip of my prosthesis.

Dr. Channon first stated the complexities of Inflammatory Breast Carcinoma. Then he suggested three drug regimens not aforementioned in your office:

1. Taxotere

2. 5FU—a continuous low-dose infusion

3. Herceptin lottery study

His lab technician started Her2Neu testing necessary to qualify for the Herceptin study; but we all agreed there is no time to fool around waiting to be accepted. My needs are immediate.

At the end of our session, Channon favored Taxotere. "Let's begin Taxotere and get this thing settled down." I grabbed hold of his matter-of-fact statement like my life depended on it. A positive image popped up: inflamed malignancy settling down. My life does depend upon this. Okay. Let's go!

Connie

Tuesday, June 3, 1997

Hello Wizard of Medicine:

Thanks for not wasting time implementing Dr. Channon's suggestion to start the drug Taxotere. I understand FDA approved Taxotere six months ago. Cutting edge of the latest fad is an anxious position for me. I am more a beaten path, tried-and-true type gal. So you've given Taxotere to only one other patient and you will not tell me how he or she is faring? Did he or she bite the dust?

But we already know Connie Titus is a different composition. It is a brand new Tuesday morning with a stronger drug and a hopeful image on the docket. I love the way God grants new starts whether we deserve them or not.

Taxotere dripped easy. My daughter, Caryn, sat beside me boosting white cells as only daughters can. You presented your body, a big smile, and thumbs up at the threshold. I whispered to myself repeatedly, "Let's start Taxotere and get this thing settled down." Visions of Dorothy from *The Wizard of Oz*[10] danced through my head.

Caryn and I left your office clicking our red, sparkly heels. We locked arms, imitating Dorothy and friends, singing and skipping down the yellow brick road to healing. My daughter has come to expect just about anything from her mom, and she is game. Patients in the parking lot were not too sure, though.

I believe with all my heart, within two weeks, we will see the skin inflammation settled down. And when it happens, I will hip-hop into your office unannounced, stand in your hallway, lift my shirt, and flash you the improvements. It will be the best offer you get all day long. Get ready to blush.

Darn. What am I doing? I just spoiled your surprise.

Taxotere is my friend.

Connie

Tuesday, June 10, 1997

Hi (a weak hi):

Taxotere my friend—phooey! Thanks for seeing me in your Holly Hill office yesterday. Two elderly church friends cancelled their doctors' appointments to drive me southwest. We got lost in a summer downpour, horns honked on all sides. But I needed you, wherever, especially after Sunday's emergency-room visit. Please know I am thinking over your advice to buck up, suck it up, and take the drugs. I need to practice compliance and submission in your care. Neal waits patiently for this too.

Maybe you and I did not thoroughly discuss Taxotere's side effects of combustion and disintegration. Otherwise I might have steered clear of the emergency room (ER).

Or was it my turn to evaluate Lawndale Hospital's ER?

You were out of town and I panicked. Every soft tissue, muscle, bone, and molecule screamed with sharp, shooting pain. In my mind it was not chemo side effects, but a grand sweep of Inflammatory Cancer, and I would expire before your return. Neupogen's painful response rated mild compared to this. I vowed aloud I would rather rot from cancer than endure this agony. What a thing to say to a loving husband who thanks me for working hard to stay alive.

For the record, the hospital, specifically the ER, is no place for sick people. The department is unsanitary (Neal stuck to the floor), inefficient (tech tried to draw the same blood test from me twice), and inattentive (I lay there for hours with no action, but that is typical of any emergency room). We walked out without walking papers. Sorry. Apologize to your partner on call, will you?

Between molecular pain and sticking to ER's floor, there has been no dancing.

My best friend since kindergarten happened to be visiting for the weekend. She creatively tried to keep an even flow throughout our household, getting our son ready for camp, soothing our daughter who didn't want to be soothed. The good news is she is still my best friend.

I will give Taxotere another consideration, supplement with pain meds, hold on tight to my responsive vision, and practice compliance, submission, and faith. Do doctors pray for patients? Dr. Collin, please say a prayer for me. Ask God to get me dancing, no matter what.

Signed,

Connie

A compliant, submissive patient,
Mrs. Connie Titus
(Neal is rolling his eyes.)

Monday, June 16, 1997

Dear Dr. Collin:

A serious illness becomes tolerable when one develops a close bond with the doctor. You and your staff are fashioning me into a personal friend of oncology. Addressing you as Alan is on the tip of my tongue, but I must maintain respect as stated in our contract.

Neal and I appreciate the time you spent with us Friday. We now understand why Dr. Cappelletti insisted upon you. Thank you for being a friend and caregiver to us both.

Saturday night something made me pick up *Dr. Susan Love's Breast Book*. Please don't make a face. Work with me. Dr. Love is a well-respected breast cancer specialist. Her Inflammatory section sounds harsh, yet I was strangely relieved to discover there are others out there. Reading about me in print fortified my immune system, at least for an evening.

I understand my first recurrence now. Dr. Love explains how Inflammatory Breast Carcinoma (IBC) involves the lymphatic vessels of the skin as well as the breast tissue. When the skin is sewn back together after a mastectomy, there is high risk for skin metastasis. For this reason, she suggests systemic treatment (chemotherapy) first, followed by local treatment (mastectomy), then radiation.

Please note I do not regret any of my decisions thus far. Dr. Love also pushes high-dose chemo coupled with Stem Cell Rescue (SCR), but she openly admits there are no statistics that SCR improves the odds. She goes on to document several different IBC cases. I cling to one of her statements. "Grim though it can be, Inflammatory Breast Cancer is still an extremely variable disease."[11]

I wish to be on the good variable team. Is it too late for me or not? I worship a God of miracles. He appears to be able.

The body of this letter is trying to convey…I don't know what the body of this letter is trying to convey. Maybe simple thanks for standing beside us, for referrals, and for bear hugs that make me melt into a puddle on the floor.

Oh, and when I get well, let's all go dancin'. If God calls me home to his dance floor, I still want you all to go dancing here on earth in celebration of my life. I have had so much pleasure and delight in my lifetime.

Love,

Connie

Connie Titus, a variable IBCer

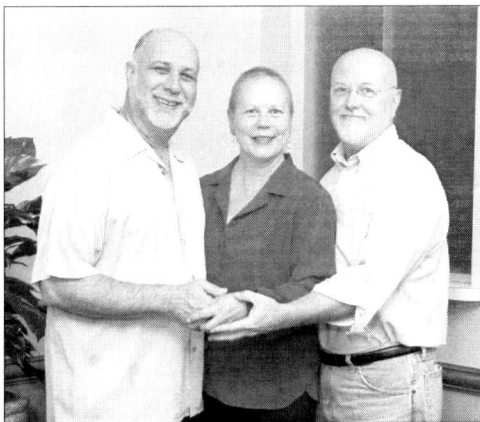

Doctor, Patient, and Husband yoke together for a three-legged race. No translation available for the two bald men, but this is what goes on behind Patient's smile. "Oh, no. My real breast is poking into the side of the professional standing beside me. Why couldn't it be my fake breast? I wouldn't even notice. But that's all I feel—the warmth—and my real breast growing bigger, bigger and bigger as we pose. Is Doctor aware? Can he hold up against warmth and rapid growth? What is he thinking? Great. Now Mr. Titus is pinching my behind. Photographer Jerry! For cryin' out loud! Take the picture!"

Courtesy of Photographer Jerry Brewer

Tuesday, June 17, 1997

Dear Medicine Man/Dance Instructor:

Taxotere is definitely my friend again. What a memorable morning appointment: unbuttoning my blouse, flashing you skin metastasis improvement, and at the same time playfully proving I can dance up a storm at daybreak, or at 10:45 a.m., whatever the case may be. Was I your first flash dance in Room #3? Be thankful your recital took place behind closed doors.

Dr. Cappelletti got his yesterday in the hallway between patients. "When was the last time a woman flashed you?" I inquired, and before he could ask what I was doing there, I lifted my top, unfastened my bra and performed a modified version of what you saw this morning. Wow, can my surgeon blush! And he's got the longest eyelashes I've ever seen on a man. Obviously, I was his best offer all day.

The last time Cappelletti inspected my chest wall, the scar line screamed with malignant inflammation. Giving us consistent bad news saddens this good man, so it tickled me to show and tell him dramatic results in unusual form. He is truly pleased and will write you a note of commendation.

The nurses and office gals squealed and hugged me too. Afterwards the blushing doctor made me tuck my shirt in, and he herded us all into the chart room for a group photo.

Mamma said there'd be days like this. Good strong hands guide my child-like body. I am ecstatic about the chain of command. God started the ball rolling by leading me to the hands of my boss and his wife, Dr. and Mrs. Greg Morrison. When trouble arose with a rather private body part, my employers passed me along into the hands of their skilled surgeon friend, Marvin J. Cappelletti. Dr. Cappelletti insisted I be handled by you and your caring bunch, and you, in turn, called in the hands and brains of four other specialists. On top of this team, there are hands offering prescriptions behind the scenes. Extraordinary professionals watch out for me, and this brings my family solace.

At this morning's recital you looked like a cross between a proud parent and a wide-eyed man at a burlesque show, the perfect audience for my only-child syndrome. Thank you. And thanks for your continued *dance* instruction. But don't expect any more flash dancing from me. That was a one-time deal. Next week I will waltz with Matilda wearing a turtleneck.

Today's flash dance makes Taxotere worthwhile. This day goes into my memory bank; how about you? I will see you for the second Taxotere treatment on June 24. I promised you submission and compliance. Please know I try.

Connie

Wednesday, July 2, 1997

Hello:

Taxotere report: Days four to eight are rough. Pains shoot through my organs, muscles, tissues, bones, and every other fiber of my being. I try to bite the bullet rather than family members or ER techs. Due to a phobia of narcotics, I abstain from taking anything that spells relief. My mouth fills up with sores and even water tastes metallic. Steroids prevent me from sleeping. Yeah, I am one broken record, a scratched 45, crackling, playing the same notes over and over again. And you, I'm sure, would like to rip me off the turntable and snap me in half. Please do so.

Dr. Collin, in your opinion, does visualization promote success in treatment? Cancer buddies tell me the importance and coax me to share their imagery.

Some patients imagine their chemo as Pacman chewing up the disease. Others visualize a Star Wars scene with speed-of-light traveling, laser beams, loud noise, etc. Still others employ soldiers who shoot, or sharks that shred the evil cells. These flicks work for many but not for me. Pacman gobbles up the cancer, becomes diseased himself, and remains in the body. How is this helpful? You are still full of disease. A Star Wars scene sounds like turmoil, an edge-of-your-seat type of process. I had enough of that in prior employment. Can you imagine the scar tissue left behind by soldiers and sharks?

Below is my rendition of chemotherapy visualization: a peaceful, spiritual approach. Refrain from yawning, please.

As Taxotere enters my infusaport, the drug transforms from liquid into a band of angel atoms marching one hundred million strong. They divide into troops. Each battalion surrounds one angular-shaped, destructive cancer cell. They join hands entrapping the culprit. The angel atoms then begin Gregorian chants.

Are you familiar with Gregorian chants? Male voices sing melodic, liturgical songs—usually in Latin. The ensemble blends in unison without accompaniment, and this takes place in monasteries, large cathedrals, or temples where acoustics are absolutely incredible. The sound is soothing, spellbinding. A few years ago Neal bought me a Gregorian Chant CD,[12] so all I have to do is pop that in and begin the imagination.

Chanting captivates and stabilizes the cancer cell, softening its frenzy. Following the chant, intense prayer is spoken until the cell drops down—humble, sorry, porous. At this time a warm, bright light radiates through the bad cell, dissolving it completely, without a trace, for all eternity.

Angel atoms rejoice, dance up a storm, and quickly seek another angular cancer cell to conquer. Reinforcements move in every twenty-one days.

Connie Titus' visualization leaves no battle scars. My body is filled with music, spiritual and physical energy and that warm, bright light—an afterglow, if you will. Lately I've been enticed into a sun dance on our eastern front porch early in the morning. Neal stands amazed, drinking his coffee, watching with a twinkle in his eye.

God himself said, "Let there be light in the darkness…" (2 Corinthians 4:6, TLB). Yes, let there be warm, bright light in my darkness.

Peace to you, Alan S. Collin, M.D.,

Connie

Thursday, July 10, 1997

Hey, Guy,

I hang on tight. The jury is still out whether Taxotere is my friend this week. I'll let you know.

Meanwhile, can we revisit the self-image issue?

Join me in a favorite daydream. I am seated in your office for a post treatment check-up. No blue paper gowns from the drawer this time. I wear a fitted jacket, low-cut colorful camisole, short skirt, sheer sexy nylons, and high heels. A head full of dark, short, curly hair is my most striking feature. Eye makeup enhances real eyebrows, real eyelashes. Unique jewelry adorns my healed, tanned neckline and completes a dazzling effect.

You walk in with a double take. Who is this woman? For a split second you are just a man, gazing. Say goodbye to that sad, overweight, bald blob of a patient and hello to an attractive, sensual woman. Hometown folks acknowledge me as a lusty, healthy, outspoken, and self-confident woman suitable to run for any office. Resuming my old life with gusto and exploring brand new opportunities definitely contribute to the glow you feast your eyes upon.

You are cute as just a man, gazing.

"We are such stuff as dreams are made on…"[13]

Back to present day filled with hindsight. I never really appreciated my God-given feminine curves. I did not take time to admire the beauty of my breasts, explore their sensitivity, or dress them up fancy. Tattered, faded bras were good enough for me. I could have at least ordered from Victoria's Secret for Neal's pleasure. Now it's too late.

I've taken other body parts for granted too. I was not one to manicure or polish healthy nails. Now their stains, ugly ridges, and brokenness drive me crazy. Before cancer I had really nice legs. A girlfriend at the citrus plant would comment, "Best legs in town!" But lately the best legs in town retain fluid and could easily explode under pressure while dancing at daybreak. Four-course meals brought in by church ladies contoured a huge, rippling behind, but I must eat and not hurt their feelings, yes? My shoulders hunch forward from heavy burdens and I've adopted a poor, lopsided attitude. The left arm swells. Various head coverings are hot, scratchy, and bothersome. I hate them and look vicious because of it. Bloodshot eyes and dark circles from tear-stained nights add a perfect touch to this real mirror image. Are you having fun at my pity party? It's my party, I *will* cry if I want to.

According to the American Cancer Society, surviving women take more interest in personal care. I should start now, fuss over myself, and summon up a tiny bit of magnetism. But why? I forget why.

Did I ever show you the photo below? Take off your stethoscope. Be a man. Gaze.

• • •

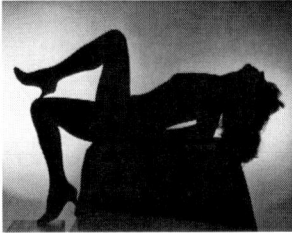

Patient Connie, before cancer, living a charmed life. Prior to carving, shaving, and steroid weight gain, a boudoir photo session pampered Connie into a Victoria's Secret role model.

Courtesy of Photographer Ed Staten

• • •

Alan S. Collin, M.D., beware of breast cancer gals obsessed with vanity. I tease you about being vain, but we are allowed, or are we? See what God says about vanity.

> Don't be concerned about the outward beauty that depends on jewelry, or beautiful clothes, or hair arrangement. Be beautiful inside, in your hearts, with the lasting charm of a gentle and quiet spirit which is so precious to God.
>
> 1 Peter 3:3-4 (TLB)

Love from a vain daydreamer,

Connie

Connie

Wednesday, July 16, 1997

Good Evening,

Neal and I just love you. Thank you for yesterday's high-quality office visit. You calmed us, made us laugh, empowered us, took the pressure off, cleared our heads, and bear-hugged me. (Neal passes on bear hugs.) We both emerged with hope.

As I marched to the exit with my allotment of hope, I noticed your waiting room bursting at the seams. The natives were restless, each one desperate for hope.

A scenario came to mind. Is this a typical day in the life of Alan S. Collin, M.D.?

You spend a tumultuous morning trying to catch up, a lost cause. At 2:07 p.m. you force down half a dry sandwich and a warm Coke. An over-booked afternoon begins, ready or not. The evening's hospital run is chaotic. You and your heartburn arrive home very late. Your first inclination is to slam doors, kick the dog, snap at the wife and kids...until you open the front door of your house. Oh, no. There they are. The wife and kids are lined up on the sofa, all dressed up with no place to go. You've forgotten about dinner with the neighbors. You look in the direction of the household bar to see barely a teaspoon in your beloved Scotch bottle. You offer yet another clumsy apology. Exhausted, you stumble up the stairway muttering, "Don't touch me. Don't talk to me. Don't look at me."

I wish I could whisper assurance in your ear that all your agonizing effort matters to patients like me.

Who takes care of the caregivers—doctors, nurses, counselors? You all give and give to thankless jobs (and read quirky letters) receiving little in return. Working for a surgeon makes me slightly more sensitive to a doctor's demands. While our boss is giving considerable time doing the hope thing, we girls pace back and forth in the hallway, so close to pounding on the door with a plea, "Could you hurry up in there, please? Don't you know there is standing room only in the waiting room, and oh, by the way, patients in examining rooms #2 and #3 have either developed gangrene or committed hara-kiri with the instruments." By the day's end, our boss is fed up. So are we.

Under the influence of cancer, questions run through my beady little mind concerning your complicated business of oncology. How does a young medical student choose a career where life and death stage a constant battle? Did your academic textbooks indicate that a starched white coat is an emotional shield? Forget that! Do professors lecture on what to expect inside cancer clinic cubicles? Do interns take turns squinting through clinical peepholes or monitoring overhead audio/video equipment to get necessary insight? Uh oh. Now I need to scout for your hidden microphones.

Who knows how a good doctor, especially an oncologist, finds any balance between work and play? Maybe I hang around to intercede. I hereby write you a prescription to move you in that direction. Dr. Collin, balance is an attainable factor in your life. With this prescription in hand, figure it out.

Connie B. Titus, I.B.C.P.
151 Windemere Drive Ormond Beach, FL 32104 987-654-3210

Name: Alan S. Collin, M.D., P.A.
Address: 2100 Nottingham Avenue, Suite #107
Date: 7/16/97

Rx: Take as directed by Mrs. Charles Cowman in *Streams in the Desert*: [Excerpts] "…calm retreat…silent shade… quiet musing…do nothing, think nothing, plan nothing… As often as you can, get away from the fret and fever of life, into fields. Wearied with the heat and din, the noise and bustle, communion with nature is very grateful; it will have a calming healing influence. A walk through the fields, or a saunter by the seashore...will purge your life of sordidness and make the heart beat with new joy."[14]

Also prescribed: sit beside your wife on the veranda at sunset. Sing a song. Earth, Wind & Fire offers some great suggestions in their tune "Sing a Song": "When you feel down and out, sing a song; here's a time to shout, sing a song; give yourself what you need, sing a song; smile, smile, smile and believe, sing a song."[15]

I thought about attaching your official-looking prescription to a bottle of Scotch, but chose something easier on your liver—*Billy Joel Easy Piano Collection.*[16] So, after you sing a song on the veranda, go inside and tickle the ivories. Maybe Jeanne will dance for you, if you ask her *nicely.*

You once told me immune systems are strengthened by music and dancing. You, of all people, need a substantial dose. See what you can do, buddy. I'll check your pulse next week.

With compassion,

Connie

Connie

Sunday, July 20, 1997

Chief:

Apparently a neighbor saw me at the mailbox with my rug on. Our neighborhood presented us with a generous bag of money along with a note suggesting I should *please* buy a decent-looking wig. Hmm. Was I that scary?

I agree. My mail-order wig is where the term rug comes from. It is fashioned much like my short haircut before chemotherapy; however, it does not fit right. The darned thing is uncomfortable, too thick, and, well, downright comical.

Thursday morning I drove downtown to Allison's Wig Shoppe to see if I could find a professional hairpiece—a sexy style that would please the neighbors, the mailman, Neal, and me and you. I tried on brunette wigs, blond wigs, natural gray wigs, and redhead wigs in all styles and lengths.

Every time I put on a blond wig, I thought of you. I've watched you, Mr. Obvious, walking through the chemo room when there are blond women in there—your head jerks back and forth like you're watching a tennis match. Brunettes, grays, redheads could flag you down with a real problem and you wouldn't even notice. Now that I think about it, most of your nurses and staff members are blond. Evidently I need to be blond to get your attention. Blond it is.

There's a man in Holly Hill that specializes in thinning and styling wigs. He worked me in Thursday afternoon. All wigs come with way too much hair. He did a nice job on this one. Looks natural, yes?

My sister, Judy, often accompanies me to oncology appointments, but you'll never meet her. I won't allow her to come into the cubicle. Do you know why? She is a sexy blond. If she were in the room with us, you wouldn't hear one single word out of my mouth. Your eyes would be fixed on her and you'd respond to me making no sense whatsoever. For example, if I were complaining of pain, you'd say, "Oh, Connie, you are in pain? That is very nice. What color is it?"

Grrr.

Funny, Neal used to be sweet on nothing but brunettes. Now he's swinging over to blonds. What is it with gray-haired men digging blonds?

How did I look on Friday? You made a favorable comment about my wiggle down the hallway, but did I smell like a blond?

Later dude,

Connie

Connie

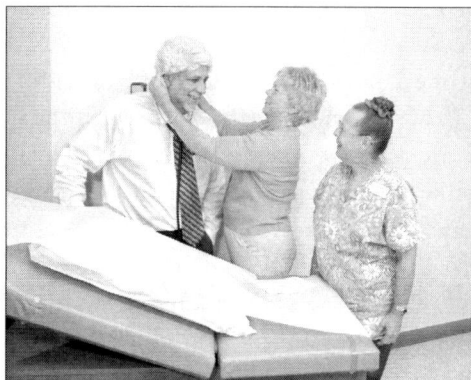

Nurse Alice and Patient Connie attempt to style the Chief's goofy wig.

Courtesy of Photographer Jerry Brewer

Tuesday, July 22, 1997

Dear Alan S. Collin, M.D.,

Three Taxotere treatments are notched on my belt. I can't decide if I am choking or taking charge. What's your opinion?

Some days I feel halfway normal and it is hard to believe I am sick. Other days nagging pain, sheer exhaustion, or a glimpse of my bald, naked body chokes all normalcy right out of me.

Last weekend Neal and I retreated for a much-needed getaway. I hoped to go dancing, but most of all I wanted to lounge around the hotel pool in my flat, blue swimsuit. Prosthesis and wig were not necessary because no one knew me or cared. My loving husband accompanied me to the pool.

The process of relaxation became disturbed, however, when whole, healthy female bodies pranced by, singly or in groups, right in front of us. It was like watching some high-priced fashion show. And why couldn't they slither seductively into the water over at the far corner? Why did they have to bend over *at the waist* and dive in right in front of my husband's hungry eyes? As I type this, I can hear you asking, "Why didn't you invite me?" (How does one growl in a letter? Insert one loud growl, here.) I wanted to choke and drown every one of them, including Neal (and now you.) Will I get over this? At what age will physical flaws no longer matter?

The Radiation Center is offering a free, six-week course on how to take charge of my physical and emotional health. I signed up, primed and ready. Curriculum includes stress management, relaxation, visualization, goal setting, diet, nutrition, exercise, and the importance of a positive attitude—all from a Christian viewpoint. It is a proven fact that those who maintain a positive, active approach to any disease live twice as long. Yeah. Teach me how!

Nothing is easy, though, you know? The class meets at night when my energy level cannot be calculated. It is late when I get home, and poor night vision makes finding my way in the dark a challenge for me and for other motorists. The thermometer in the Radiation Center is locked on freezing. I guess what cancer cells they can't kill with nuclear energy, they freeze. One more thing: A nice lady, whom I love, sits next to me wearing heavy perfume that chokes me and gives me a headache every time. How do I score in the positive attitude section?

Along with taking charge of my own healthcare, I take charge of other women's healthcare. Do you know what my daytime job is? I schedule Dr. Morrison's surgeries. That means I arrange for other women to have their breasts cut off.

Last Thursday was a day from down under. I reported for work despite a sleepless night. Darvocet and Coca Cola was the breakfast of this champion. With dark, puffy bags under my eyes and my uniform buttoned crooked, I stepped off the elevator as one gruesome sight. We faced a full docket of patients that day. Dr. Morrison instructed me to schedule not one, not two, but three mastectomies. Can you believe it? Our town suffers a rash of breast cancer. Am I contagious?

Let me briefly explain what happens when a mastectomy survivor schedules the same surgery for another woman. The surgeon ushers his stunned breast cancer patient to my desk. She is ghostly white. She is either alone or with a helpmate, who is also white as a ghost. We all sit down together. The patient faces me, at the edge of my desk. I fight to maintain color in my face.

First, I must start the frustrating task of insurance clearance or payment plans. Why this uncomfortable issue must be handled first and done with the shocked, pitiful patient sitting right in front of me, I'll never know. We might as well hammer the first nail into her coffin. If or when that unfair red tape is in place, my fingers do the walking over to our hospital's outpatient department where pre-testing appointments and the surgery date and time are scheduled.

The telephone receiver is glued to my head for at least thirty minutes during which time the patient and/or her helpmate have ample time to run away. For those who stay, I dry tears, I switch to speakerphone and steady them on the way to the ladies' room where some of them upchuck, and I reach out with a warm hand and understanding eyes as best I can. But their labored breathing and racing heartbeats bring me back to just yesterday when I was that pale, sad woman at the edge of a scheduling desk. God chokes me with the reality.

At some point I snap back. I gather the patient's appointment schedules, instructions, and blessed hospital policies, top it off with a pretty little blue-and-white booklet explaining the mastectomy surgical procedure, and secure it all with a shiny silver paperclip shaped like an angel. Slowly I walk the patient through our waiting room and out our front door. And then what do I say? Have a nice day? Thank you for shopping at Dr. Morrison's? Don't forget to read our money-back guarantee?

I don't know how, on that particular day, I was able to pull it off three times—*bam, bam, bam*—without upchucking myself. But I did, by God's good grace. I poured out all the encouragement I could manage.

This job is a supreme test and purpose for me. Most days I look at it as an opportunity to offer life jackets for those in the same boat. When my white cells are sufficient and I feel determined, I visit patients in the hospital. I make myself available by phone for answering questions and openly share ways of nurturing the body. Neal worries about me. He says I'm too close to the problem.

He may be right. But for now, this is where I serve.

Signed,

Connie

Connie Titus, Your Friendly Mastectomy Coordinator

Thursday, July 31, 1997

Hey! Dr. Collin!

I picked up a *Garfield* card for you today. It looks like someone just drop-kicked *Garfield*. He's all sprawled out in a sad manner. The expression on his face is a perfect replica of me on Tuesday. Sad *Garfield* expresses, "Sometimes when I feel like nobody understands me, it helps to think of you." Then you open the card and he says, "Nobody understands you either!"[17] Ha. My sentiments exactly.

Even though I don't understand you, I do love you. Loving you allows me to be frank. You ticked me off, and I have the guts to tell you.

For three or four days my pain-riddled body and emotionally crippled soul suffered sleep deprivation. Yes, much of it is self-induced due to my fear of taking addictive, prescribed meds, but it's easier to blame you. I shuffled around behind you through the hallway, whimpering and bellyaching, and then I caught a glimpse of my friend Nanette Barrish (pretty, petite, tan Nanette), taking her Taxotere like a trooper. How embarrassing. I must have looked utterly foolish to both of you.

What I desperately needed from my doctor, sir, was one of your tender verbal strokes. "I am sorry you are feeling bad," "You are doing good hard work," or "I am very proud of you." Was this too much to ask?

Instead, you whirled around, positioned your face to within one inch of my face, and growled. "Connie! Addictive or not, you have no choice but to take these drugs right now. If you have an addiction problem, we will fix it later."

Were you in the Army?

I cried all the way home, but swallowed the drugs and thankfully got a decent night's sleep. God arranged for a valuable lesson to permeate my soul and fill my mind at daybreak.

Whether you meant to or not, the valuable lesson I learned is how *not* to rely on your assurance and your touch. Yes, pampering is nice, but I must practice independence from humans and depend only on the Lord. His pampering is sufficient. Better yet, I should forget about myself and let God have his way with me. "…learn to put aside your own desires so that you will become patient and godly, gladly letting God have his way with you" (2 Peter 1:6, TLB).

Learning and applying what I've learned are two different things, and frankly, way too much to ask right now.

Bottom line: thanks for the kick in the pants. You are molding my sassy rear-end. From what I gather, the compliant, weak, and needy patient doesn't fare as well, or as long, as the active, self-sufficient, occasionally sassy patient.

But wait, back up, let me tell you one more weak and needy thing before I cross over. I hate to be suspended on drugs. I have no idea who I am, who I was, who I want to be, or if any of it matters. My mother died as a result of prescription narcotics eating away at her organs. I wrestle with a justified drug phobia. In the future, a slight bit of compassion will be sincerely appreciated.

Would it be easier if patients enter the clinic carrying a banner listing moods, needs, and exactly how we expect you to interact? No. You are right, poor idea. We are here to talk with the doctor, not a robot. You've mentioned feeling like a mechanical robot on occasion, and you don't like it much. Okay, no prompting necessary.

I am contemplating the next treatment and how I might help myself. Ideally I want to build a hibernation cave, refusing to see anyone, including you. My cave resembles an Amish cabin with hardwood floors furnished only with a single bed, one straight chair, and a roughly sawn cedar table. The ocean breeze blows lace curtains over an open Bible. Early morning sunbeams coax me into a polka, all by myself.

Today starts a new week. We are all thrilled with my outward response to Taxotere. Yet maybe I'm still a young woman facing a shortened life span. There are certain things I wish to accomplish.

I replay your voice suggesting: "One day at a time, Connie. Healing comes first. Accomplishments will fall into place. Meanwhile, dance!"

Thanks again for the drop kick. I trust you will let me know if I become a pain-in-the-rear-end patient.

Love,

Connie

Connie, a sassy patient with a dent in her rear-end *matching your shoe size.*

Wednesday, August 6, 1997

Doctor, Captain, Director:

Bed rest ushers my brain to new horizons. I just turned up the volume on my imagination.

You are directing and producing a science fiction movie and I am the star. Lucky me.

My Character Profile

Taxotere treatments one through four are done and over with. Side effects accumulate. The plus side: there is little or no nausea, no fever, and no emergency-room inspection in the last seven weeks. I do, though, suffer through four or five sleepless nights in a row due to steroids. Pain shoots through my organs, tissues, muscles, and bones. My ears ache, my nose bleeds, my mouth is full of sores, and a thick coating on the tongue makes even water taste disgusting. Concentrated discomfort throbs in the mastectomy area, shoulders, and neck. My neck feels as if someone is choking me. Bloating presses on my rib cage; an explosion may be near. Call me a recluse; a hermit I am. Shampoo commercials cause extreme aggravation. Our bathroom mirror reflects a distorted, sick, painful-looking blob. Planting flowers and riding waves is over—forever. I neglect my family when I'm not altering their lifestyles. I have no idea what is needed to help. There is no end in sight, no comfort, no peace.

My husband says you, Dr. Collin, have created a monster, not a star.

Scenario

Ormond-By-The-Sea's oncology office opens for one hour on weekends and holidays for patients needing Neupogen shots or blood chemistries. A sad scene: good, innocent folks shuffle in to be shot up with chemicals. Most don't know what drugs or dosages they are getting. We are no longer humans. We are mannequins presenting ourselves for puncture wounds while you play golf. Sorry—a hit below your belt. Won't someone please pick us up and set us firmly in place with purpose and strength?

"After you have suffered a little while, our God, who is full of kindness through Christ, will give you his eternal glory. He personally will come and pick you up, and set you firmly in place, and make you stronger than ever" (1 Peter 5:10, TLB).

• • •

Alan S. Collin, M.D., P.A., the golfing doctor, captain of many ships, director of this science fiction film: Whew! You are a busy fellow. You and I engage to fight this battle. There are many demands upon your time. If you divvy out hope to each patient as you do with me, you are stretched too thin. However, I am greedy. This type of personal danger has never crossed my path before. How can I get you to hold my hand on a daily basis? No pressure. It is my childhood complex speaking. Remember, I need to establish strong contact with the teacher/director.

I will come in next week to inform other patients to step back. "Step away from the Doctor. He belongs to me. I am the star of his show."

Signed:

Connie

Connie, The Star of Your Show…a dancing star. Even with the above profile, I am mastering the Mazurka, a Polish folk dance in three-quarter time. Not at daybreak, though. More like mid-afternoon.

Monday, August 11, 1997
Hand-Delivered To Anybody Who Cares.

Dr. Collin, would that be you?

It is me. Connie Titus #25561. I am crying for attention.

You want me to take another treatment tomorrow? I can't. I am on the edge. "Why?" you ask. I'll tell you why. How many reasons do you need?

I suffer aggressive breast cancer and have had six months of aggressive chemotherapy. I face radiation and possibly more chemo. An early death looms.

Chemicals saturate me. They supposedly eat the bad cells, but they also eat my soul. My spirituality, my common sense, my very being is swallowed up. Drug-induced menopause is here. My family is fearful.

While opening the closet to store cancer, all my past problems, sins, and secrets come tumbling out. Broken pieces, spills, and stains lie everywhere. It is a mess. It is hopeless. I am hopeless.

Certain needs drive me to drink. I have urgent needs before I check out. No one understands. No one can meet these needs. I am trapped in a bald, overweight, deformed body no man would find attractive. Even my personality is no longer desirable.

Because of my craze, I hide from God, which is ridiculous. He records my craze before it happens.

What about all those people who send continuous cards and meals? They address me as brave, faithful, and pure. Oh, what foolish friends.

Screw your dancing at daybreak idea.

Okay. It is written and proclaimed that I can offer God anything and he will straighten it out. I can give him each messy entry above and pray he still loves me.

Please still my storm, dear Lord. Bring me out of desperation.

"Then they cried out to the Lord in their trouble, and he brought them out of their distress. He stilled the storm to a whisper; the waves of the sea were hushed" (Psalm 107:28-29, NIV).

Doctor, I suppose you will call me this afternoon with your famous "you can do it" speech. Please be gentle. I am vulnerable, laid wide open. Tomorrow might be brighter. Who knows? I could have a whole new attitude by morning—come bee-bopping in for a cocktail right after I dance the Highland Fling with my niece out by the tree house. Or maybe I should call the shrink. In that case, I'll see you next Tuesday.

Love from someone teetering on the edge. And that could be any one of your four-hundred ninety-three patients, so I will identify myself:

Connie

Connie Beth Thompson Titus
#25561

Thursday, August 21, 1997

Doctor, Sir:

Golly. Stumbling and falling through the last portion of this regimen is embarrassing. For eight months I've maintained a stiff upper lip, displayed stamina and dignity and defied IBC odds by wearing a uniform and reporting to work. That is something to be proud of. The young cancer/chemo patients who file through Dr. Morrison's office have all applied for disability. But at last, I succumb to being a sick, out-of-commission chemo patient. May I act the part now?

How can I love you so deeply and be convinced you are trying to kill me at the same time? Tuesday you tried to kill me with Neupogen. Come on. You know how I twist and shout with the side effect of severe bone pain, yet you ordered a higher dose. Do I have a low tolerance for pain? No. I am just super-sensitive to the drug. A full syringe is way too much. Agreed, I needed a white-count boost, but I begged and cried for a lower dose. Nurse Molly explained you were protecting me from harm's way.

Later that day I proceeded to make myself sick on Tylenol #3. Then my left arm went completely numb, for no reason, which really startled me.

Yesterday, Nurse Molly, with syringe in hand, called me back to the chemo room for a second high-dose shot. Neal and I held her captive in the waiting room and made her squirt a bit onto the carpet (probably $149.95 worth). We told her we were willing to sign a form releasing her from your reprimand.

Important note: What squirt onto the floor was the drug from the syringe. This letter reads like Neal and I squeezed Nurse Molly so tight that *she* squirted onto the floor!

Medically, I wish I could compare myself to some other real person. I seem to be your only Inflammatory patient who received and failed three Adriamycin treatments followed by four Taxotere treatments. Those are two tough drugs. I have suffered and supposedly conquered a recurrence midstream and am still alive to tell about it. The fact that I have not fallen into the pot with other statistics is kind of neat, but could I gain recognition by some other means such as sparkling personality, intense spirituality, or creative penmanship? For someone with a real phobia of prescription drugs and chemicals, and not at all liking to be on the cutting edge, Connie Titus has just accomplished the impossible.

Early on I made a deal with God. I promised him I would accept pain, hair loss, humility, insanity, mouth sores, insomnia, menopause, hot flashes, headaches, and other heartaches that come with the cancer package if only he would protect me from nausea and vomiting. I hate to vomit. In the last eight months, I can count on one hand the number of nausea episodes. God graciously keeps up his end of the deal. I, though, fall short. This last month you've heard me complain aloud, sob, and writhe because Connie Titus may never, among other things, hit another flea market on Saturday mornings.

What I need to do is revisit my initial choice of conventional chemotherapy here at home. By doing so I will again count all my blessings, which include: loving, gentle doctors and nurses who believe in treating the whole person; the comfort of my home, my cave; understanding family and friends who nourish me with food and prayer daily; generous employers who provide me with purpose, encouraging me to do what I can, when I can; occasional replicas of the normal me as mom, housewife, and child of God.

With that said and done, I feel better. I might even kick up my heels while praising God. I have much joy in my life, even during this life-threatening hullabaloo.

Instead of reprimanding Nurse Molly for squirting Neupogen onto your waiting room carpet, thank her, please. My skeleton is intact because of her willingness. Neal and I will arrange for the carpet to be steam-cleaned. I hope we did not cause a chain reaction with other patients.

Signed,

Connie

Connie

P.S. Have I told you lately I love you? I'm telling you now. I love you.

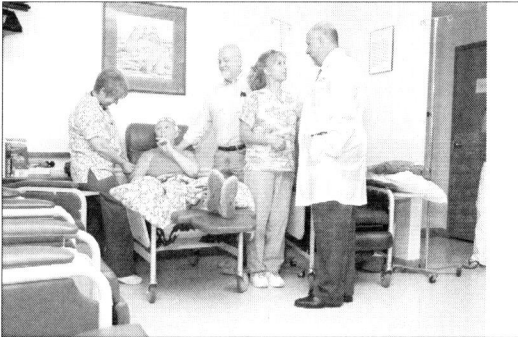

Nurse Molly, Patient Connie, and Husband Neal shush each other and whisper over the fact that part of Connie's expensive Neupogen shot soaks into the waiting room carpet. Nurse Nicole distracts Dr. Collin from discovering their secret.

Courtesy of Photographer Jerry Brewer

Friday, September 5, 1997

Dear Doctor:

Ten reasons for me to cry, and I do.

1. Hair: The hair I proudly grew back after first treatment falls out again. Doggone it.

2. Rejection: With your referral, I paid a visit to Johanson Sports Medicine. A massage called Manual Lymph Drainage should reduce the Lymphadema in my left arm. After an in-depth interview and examination, they thought it too dangerous. Fluid to be moved contains bacteria and debris that could aggravate Inflammatory Carcinoma. Plus the lymph nodes they normally move the fluid to will soon be radiated. Johanson's therapist declined her services. Also, I told psychiatrist Dr. Rigel I could no longer afford him. Insurance only pays $20.00 of his $150.00/hr. fee. Could he work a deal with me? Oh, no. He promptly pulled out his phone book searching for a therapist on a lower level, like he couldn't wait to get rid of me.

3. Resentment: A co-worker resents everything I say or do. My employers want me to oversee their front office. I fight to save my life while running an office. Why should I subject myself to resentment on a daily basis?

4. Radiation phobia: Radiation is about to begin. I am afraid. Lying on a cold, hard table under a massive machine with no other human nearby does not sound good. It is an assault of a different nature. Do you think I can accomplish this and remain cheerful?

5. Disappointment: No trip to Ohio in October for me. No autumn, no OSU band, no family reunion. When, God, when? Or the real question is, will I ever?

6. Hot flashes: I am on fire at least once an hour. My face, scalp, neck, and gradually the whole body burns and sweats bullets, a sick panicky experience. You men. You miss out.

7. Parenting: Where are my parenting skills? Ron is not doing well in school. I regard this as a personal failure.

8. Distention of abdomen: By evening my abdomen looks like seven months of pregnancy. Is it fluid or gas? Whatever. I am extremely uncomfortable.

9. Chemicals: It might take me six weeks to rid myself of your pesky chemotherapy drugs. Sorry if I sound critical.

10. Emotion: I cry or wail at least once a day on the closet floor. It's my secret place for praying to and pleading with God the Father. "…when you pray, go away by yourself, all alone, and shut the door behind you and pray to your Father secretly…" (Matthew 6:6, TLB). It can't be too secretive because I wail rather loudly.

• • •

"Why wear a frown? Where's your faith now?" you ask. Please hang in there, Dr. Collin. Hopefully God will tough it out too, forgiving his child, Connie Titus, who looks on the bleak side today.

There is no need for you to respond. File this list of woes under, "Breast Cancer Mind in Action." Other patients might like to know they have company. You can whip my letter out and comfort them.

Marissa said she brought in a citrus box to store my letters. The box sits on the third shelf in your office. Normal procedure is to bind a patient's personal greetings in his or her chart, but since I am not and never will be a candidate for normal procedure, I accept my position of honor in a citrus box on your shelf.

Signed,

Connie

One bleak, lopsided Connie Titus

P.S. Someone notified the radio station about my complaints. WQSC played "Mighty Might" for me on the way to work this morning. I'll tell you what: Earth, Wind & Fire can take a bleak, cryin' attitude and make it into something sexy. I turned them up full blast and boogied as much as one can in the driver's seat of a Grand Marquis at the Olantangy Road/ 9th Street intersection. People stared with their mouths open. My whole car rocked. Dr. Collin, what I want to know is— what *am* I gonna do 'bout my living thang, besides dance?

Walk around, why wear a frown…

…How's ya faith? Cause ya faith is you…

We are people of the Mighty…

What ya gonna do? 'Bout your living thang?

Will ya make it better, or just complain?

Every day is real, don't run from fear

'Cause better days are very near

There are times when you are bound to cry

One more time, head to the sky.[18]

Monday, October 20, 1997

My Dear M.D. (My Doctor):

Five weeks of radiation are crossed off my calendar. Office visits with you are few during this segment. I trust you are maintaining good humor.

Say, you are a newly married man, aren't you? What I am about to share may shape your husbandry.

Birthdays, anniversaries, and holidays keep happening even though I am sick. Twenty-four years ago today my husband answered, "I do, in sickness and in health." Oh, the irony of it all. If you ask Neal, we've actually been married forty-eight long, hard, grueling years—twenty-four for him plus twenty-four for me. I try to convince folks *and Neal* that seasons of wedded bliss are tucked in there…somewhere.

There will be no celebrative wining, dining, dancing, or romance tonight. My radiated chest wall prefers not to wear a bra/prosthesis or move around too much. Instead, we will observe our special day alone with quiet honor and appreciation, right here in our humble abode where there isn't even anything exciting in the refrigerator.

Behold a "picture" of this year's anniversary party: Neal tells his annual story of how my Mom drew up a contract and paid him a lump sum to get me out of the house. She died before he could amend that contract, and believe me, he wanted to. *Yada, yada, yada (*embellishment on last year's rendition). After that's out of the way, we will probably eat a grilled cheese sandwich by candlelight at our kitchen table, exchange cards, and settle down to watch TV. Is that sad, or what? I could at least muster a kiss, a smile, and a prayer of thanksgiving after all his time and trouble. Mr. Titus really deserves a big sparkling jewel in his crown.

Our twenty-fourth year of marriage has been a mind-boggling year. My husband never knows what he'll find when he comes home at night. I can be sobbing uncontrollably, the next minute laughing, dancing, or shouting. This is very unsettling for he who witnesses, especially if it's all coming together in one hour. Ecclesiastes 3:11 states that everything is appropriate in its own time. There you go. My behavior is appropriate.

Last Wednesday was breakdown day. Why do I keep driving myself over to the Radiation Center for more abuse? The area being zapped burns like blue blazes. Not just topical pain—it is a deep-down tissue pain and I am conscious of it with every breath. Two weeks ago I told people radiation is a piece of cake compared to chemo. I retract that statement.

Pain coupled with fear of "what if" bears down hard. I am close to being done with everything—all treatments. Then what? My future is uncertain. God whispers, "Yoo Hoo, Connie. Every human's future is uncertain. You are no different." To which I have no problem arguing, "Hush, Lord, yes I am."

When my gray-bearded caregiver walked through the door Wednesday evening, loud wailing (with sackcloth) horrified him. He suffered that supreme sensation of helplessness. By the way, Neal asked me who wrote your little caregiver's guide defining his position as *helper?* There is no way to help or soothe me in this condition.

An hour later, wailing complete, a look of relief and composure reshaped my red face. I shed the sackcloth (ratty ol' teeshirt) and dressed in my Hawaiian shirt. I then bounded out the door for choir practice leaving this pitiful man behind to deal with his sadness.

My beloved husband repeats to himself, *Wedded bliss? Baloney!*

Yet every morning he comes to me and softly whispers how pretty I am. He assures me I am doing hard work and he is proud of me. He tells me he loves me and misses me. He misses me because I am lost and restless most of the time, and I sleep in the other end of the house so as not to disturb his sleep. I miss me, too. What happened to Neal's attractive, fun, happy, healthy bride?

This husband of mine with his early-morning tenderness is full of the fruit of the Spirit Paul talks about in Galatians 5:22.

You may not know Paul or the Spirit, so let me explain. The fruit of the Spirit is love, joy, peace, patience, faithfulness, gentleness, and self-control. If a man and wife practice such virtues throughout their long, hard, grueling years together, God guarantees a better chance of wedded bliss. Watch for it carefully, though. Bliss can hide where you least expect it, even inside a wailing, laughing, dancing, or shouting roommate.

Neal could write a book about his unpredictable roommate. What makes him stick around for twenty-four years? Helen Reddy's lyrics fit Neal: "You and me against the world…others turn their backs and walk away, but you can count on me to stay…"[19] Dr. Collin, you of all people know how many men turn their backs and walk away from one-breasted women. Neal chooses to stay. I wonder why.

Hand-in-hand it's Mr. Neal O. Titus and me against the world. We remember my initial prognosis and remain practical. At the same time, we believe our God is fully capable of miracles, even today, with no strings attached. And we see how he cares for us and protects us, today, with no strings attached. God is not just a story. He invites us to call on him.

Handing a full plate of trouble over to God and trusting him is hard for our controlling human nature, but we must. The Bible states loud and clear: "The Lord is good. When trouble comes, he is the place to go! And he knows everyone who trusts in him!" (Nahum 1:7, TLB).

Right now I need to get up from this computer chair and heat up the griddle for those grilled cheese sandwiches. Neal surfs Direct TV for mutually desirable entertainment. I will offer that man of mine a wink and a smile on my way to the kitchen.

Love from,

Connie

Connie (Neal's wailing, laughing, dancing, shouting roommate)

Tuesday, October 28, 1997

A.S.C., M.D.:

All systems reverse! I just thought of eleven reasons not to cry. Disregard my letter dated September 5.

1. Hair: Once again I have a nice, soft covering on top. In about six weeks I should be able to go out in public as myself. I found a gal trained in a program called *Look Good, Feel Better.* [20] She consulted with me on my own peach fuzz. We talked about makeup and general self-image during the recovery process. She offered good positive tools.

2. Rejection turned to acceptance: Thanks for vetoing Johanson Sports Medicine's theory. They accepted the challenge, and I have been going twice a week for Manual Lymph Drainage. My sessions are helping a great deal with pain and swelling. I wear the compression sleeve and know the exercises I should do. Insurance only allows me ten sessions, but that should get me on my way. Also, Dr. Rigel, the psychiatrist who couldn't wait to get rid of me, called to check up on me, which I thought impressive. He suggested two licensed social workers whom I'll contact once I get his bill paid off. Goofiness still floats around in my head needing validation, organization, or smoothing over. Aren't you glad that's not your department? Reading silly letters is bad enough.

3. Tension relieved: My co-worker and I are getting along better. It could be a cycle problem, hers or mine. Tension, for the time being, has been relieved.

4. Radiation in progress: I was really anxious about radiation. I didn't study this therapy like I did chemo. Everyone at the center is personable. Dr. R. K. scheduled me for thirty-eight treatments ending November 5. I could go into much detail, but you get their reports. I will tell you

that I am burnt to a crisp—blistering, peeling, and beet red. I contemplated skipping the last week of zaps, but church people are driving me. One more time I remind myself that I chose this treatment, and Neal and I are thankful for options here at home.

5. Plans to travel: After I graduate radiation, the first thing I must do is visit Ohio. I plan a ten-day sabbatical. The family stays at home. I will sleep, read, and walk bundled up. Oh, yeah, and I will think. Neal cringes when I think, so he is thankful to stay behind. Hopefully my body will rejuvenate enough to work full time with Dr. Morrison upon my return. November in Ohio will be gray and cold, but beautiful to me.

6. Menopause/hot flashes: My gynecologist started me on a natural progesterone cream, which seems to tame hot flashes. They are not as often or severe.

7. Parenting skills: As parents, all we can do is guide with love. We cannot be accountable for our child's every problem or mistake. I can still guide and love. Cancer has not yet stripped me of these two privileges.

8. Abdominal distention: The gynecologist ordered an ultrasound of the abdomen/pelvis to rule out any mass. Those results were clear. I mentioned I look like I'm pregnant. I am thankful to report I am not pregnant, but listen to Saturday night's vivid dream:

My cervix was 8.6 cm dilated. You examined me, wrote a prescription for the baby to be born in Piqua, Ohio, and promised to drive me there yourself. But an emergency called you away. Mr. Titus offered to drive me to Piqua, Ohio, if it wasn't on a Sunday because he could not forfeit any more pro-football games. I worked for a small office, and they threw a really big bash for a co-worker getting married. My pending birth paled to her social affair. She received six gifts and party hats. I only got one. I had to pee before the long birthing trip. Office personnel wouldn't let me use our restroom. They directed me to the diner next door, where there was a long line. And I could not, under any circumstance, give birth to this child until I paid Carly Henson the baby's first week of preschool tuition.

Wow! Neal declares no more Fifteen Bean Soup, Cajun Style for me.

9. Chemicals: The same chemicals I cried about, I praise. I needed harsh treatment at that time. Yes, it will be a while before they clear out of my body. My fingernails have ridges and are yellow halfway down. Once this grows out, I will be on my way to clearance.

10. Emotions: I still cry once a day, usually when the sun goes down. "… Weeping may go on all night, but in the morning there is joy" (Psalm 30:5, TLB). I am also laughing more than once a day, pacing activities, and expressing myself because Earth, Wind & Fire say I need to let my feelings show every day.[21] And my Lord says all is possible with him, so I am in good shape.

11. Jesus on board: Aunt Mary Ellen spent many years battling cancer. She gave me a tip. She said to envision Jesus beside me during the radiation zaps, working in tandem with that massive machine. So when the bull's eye is positioned, the technicians retreat, and the steel door slams shut, I begin to sing a song about the Lord being my vision and my best thought, by day and night. A soft tenor voice harmonizes with me. It's that man, Jesus of Nazareth. He is the only one allowed into such an electrifying situation. His left hand rests on my shoulder, his right hand on the machine. His beaming smile melts away any caution. Thank you, Jesus.

You are a good man for listening, Alan S. Collin, M.D. Now get back to work.

Love from,

Connie

Connie, your 8.6 cm dilated dreamer

Wednesday, November 5, 1997

Dr. Collin!

Guess what! It is finished. I did it. We did it. This morning I received a certificate of completion and walking papers from the Radiation Center.

The machine pulled away for the very last time leaving me exposed, vulnerable, and oh, so anxious. Man. Talk about hardcore emotions. Keeping with my spiritual visualization, I knew the Lord had to be in the room somewhere. But if ever I needed a tangible king to reach out and touch, it was at that moment. I whispered, "Here I am, Lord. Scoop me up in your strong arms and carry me the rest of the way. It is just you and me now. All physicians step back. Which road shall we take—the road to recovery, or another route? Don't leave me now."

The Lord and I stepped outside the door for my first breath of non-clinical, non-medicinal air.

Dr. Collin: from deep within our hearts, Neal and I thank you for seeing us through these last nine months. Yes, your drug therapies were arduous, troublesome, and cruel on occasion. But looking back with that prescribed pair of new eyes, each segment was necessary and helpful in arresting the severity of my condition. And the job was accomplished with balance because you were stern when I needed stern; funny when I needed funny; and cute, well, just generally cute all the time. That is me speaking; Neal has yet to label a man cute.

I am glad to be one of your successful Taxotere patients. It was a joint effort. My positive vision prior to the first treatment combined with your stern, funny cuteness and the prayers of mighty warriors brought this victory to fruition.

We have now done all we know to do, conventionally. When approached about what follows radiation, you stated we will stop all treatment. This is what every cancer patient waits to hear, yet ceasing fire is a frightening thought. Removing chemo tubes and pulling the radiation plug is like cutting my umbilical cord. Doctors have been spinning me around three times with surgery, chemicals, and radiation. Now you all want to shove me out the door, wave bye-bye, and *poof*— I am on my own. I will not be doing anything active to keep this beast at bay. What if I am no good on my own?

On top of that, all physicians, including you, caution me about the probability (not possibility, but probability) of recurrence. Isn't this groundwork for a negative frame of mind? Throughout this ordeal you have preached a positive attitude. Now we are expecting failure? Which is it, guys?

Sometimes God asks me the same question. "Which is it, Connie?" I go back and forth between rejoicing that he loves me so much and thinking I must have been a very bad girl. I wobble between determination and defeat. Sorry, God. At least I am honest.

Jehovah seems to remain on his throne despite fluctuation. He prepares me to go either way and considers himself the strongest, brightest thread in my triple-braided cord. In fact, *he* is my umbilical cord. Uh oh. How can I gently tell you this? You've been replaced. The strands in my triple-braided cord are Connie Beth, Neal Owen, and Jehovah Shammah, meaning the Lord is there. Don't go thinkin' you are out of the loop. The three of us love you, depend upon you, and believe in you. I hope I've conveyed that effectively in this letter.

Love,

Connie

Connie Beth *and* Neal Owen *and* Jehovah Shammah

P.S. By cutting my umbilical cord, will I flutter around aimlessly like a helium balloon losing air very fast?

Friday, November 7, 1997

Alan S. Collin, M.D.:

In one publication or another Charles F. Stanley says, "Our lives are an expression of who God is, and the way we live can have a compelling impact on the people we know."[22] Tuesday's early morning office visit was one of hope and intimacy. Your behavior had a compelling impact on a woman you know. Her name is Connie Titus.

We discussed my consistently low white-blood counts. If patients can correct anemia or low red cells by eating spinach and red meat and if we can raise potassium levels by eating bananas, then why can't we elevate white counts or immune systems by natural remedies and leave that nasty shot of Neupogen in your cupboard?

All I had to do was ask. You took me by the hand and gently led me to the front lobby. Patients looked up with intrigue and leaned into our conversation. We stood together in front of a beach scene painting. You explained that a patient can strengthen the immune system (add a few white cells) by thinking of, going to, or creating an environment of joy, beauty, serenity. What? It's that easy? Gee, thanks. The waiting room crowd thanks you too, because we all get connected to good health through your illustrations. You really do make a difference. That guiding hand was nice and warm, by the way.

The best part of Tuesday's encounter has to do with your clumsy entry. You stumbled into my cubicle looking a bit rough and spilled your coffee, for which you blamed a sleepless night. I planned to show you my latest dance, the Polonaise—a stately Polish dance—but from the looks of you, I put the recital on hold. What followed was an unexpected honor.

You described your sleepless night. After tossing and

turning until 2:30 a.m., you came down to your family room, flipped on Fox News Channel, and got caught up in an interview of two women missionaries who had been held captive in a third-world country. One woman especially conveyed a strong faith that enabled her to look beyond torture and death threats and see clearly our merciful God. You said this woman's testimony reminded you of me...*of my faith.* I was flabbergasted. No more was said about the news program. We moved on to address low blood counts, but tenderness lingered in your eyes. With a childlike, innocent expression those tender eyes seemed to whisper, "I want some of that. I want what you and that woman have."

Your comment perplexed me. On what do you base this comparison, and how do you know the degree of my faith when I don't know the degree of my faith? You and I have only been acquainted for a total of nine months. We've never talked of God, religion, or belief, until that brief moment on Tuesday.

Wait—my letters. Are you really reading my letters? You own a citrus box of them, and I guess they do reflect a small amount of my trust in God, but I never thought a busy doctor would take the time to read them, to comprehend strong faith on paper. So maybe I make a difference in your life? Is that what you are saying?

November is a good time to thank you. Thanks for your warm-handed guidance to the front lobby on a Tuesday, and thanks for stumbling into my presence that same day, trusting me enough with your innocence. And furthermore, I thank you for the possibility that my letters make a difference.

On a larger scale, tallies come in from all corners. My entire family and circle of friends are grateful I am in your care. I talk openly about my white-coated friend. They acknowledge you as one who makes a positive difference in my approach to wellness. They recognize your carriage and character as good examples, and they catch me dancing at odd times. People all around say you are what the purpose-driven life looks like. So by all means, please continue compelling impacts on Connie Titus. My survivorship is built one office visit at a time.

With appreciation,

Connie

Connie Titus

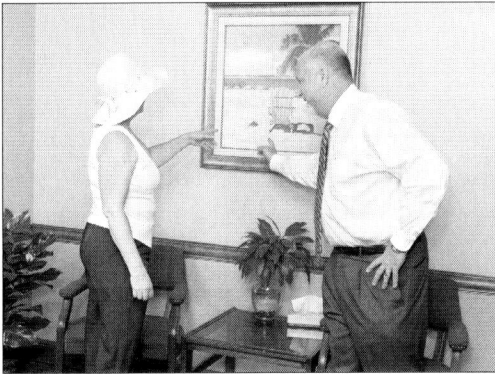

Dr. Collin describes in detail to Patient Connie how to wake up the immune system. Apparently, all you have to do is point to a beach scene painting on some wall. Any wall, any painting, really. Mind rules over matter.

Courtesy of Photographer Jerry Brewer

Monday, November 10, 1997

Dr. Alan S. Collin, M.D.:

An eerie feeling lurks. You are not expected or obligated to act on the following sensations, I am simply giving you a heads-up.

You know how a cancer patient's mind likes to talk the body into symptoms. We are overactive imaginative experts. Also, Neal thinks I have that condition/syndrome where people aren't happy unless they are in the doctor's office all the time (I forget the name of it). Other issues figure into my eeriness: a separation factor from you three physicians; the inactivity of ceasing fire; and a genuine fear that I am no good on my own. Keep all this in mind as you read.

Last Thursday I felt something new on the good (right) breast near the nipple and experienced nagging deep pain in the right armpit. Friday I had an appointment with Dr. R. K. for a post-radiation exam, so I called his attention to it. He ordered a mammogram, which read essentially normal. This morning I was concerned enough to take my films and my body to surgeon, Dr. Cappelletti. We talked awhile. He did not find or feel anything alarming. I was satisfied, yet the deep pain in the right armpit continued. If mind triumphs over matter, why can't I make this pain stop?

There is absolutely no time for nuisance or nonsense. I fly to Ohio in three days and should pack. The gnawing, doubtful, gut feeling, along with IBC research, will probably fit into my accessory bag so I can stew about it on my retreat. "Why not forget it and concentrate on relaxation and enjoyment?" Neal asks. He offered to work at solving the puzzle while I frolic. Who are we kidding? Women crave control.

My next appointment with you is November 25. I will see you then. Meanwhile, behave yourself, Alan S. Collin, M.D.

Signed,

Connie

Connie, your imaginative IBC gal

Thursday, November 27, 1997, Thanksgiving Day

Happy Thanksgiving, Friend:

How does my friend celebrate Thanksgiving? What are you thankful for? Where are you, with whom, what are you eating and talking about today? Are you at your wits' end with my inquiries and letter writing? Motion denied. If we are in business together, I need to know all about you, and you will read what I am made of inside these letters.

Neal and our son like to fish on Thanksgiving Day. My daughter and I have been upright in the kitchen for hours putting together a big turkey spread for a small group. I insist on making three dishes that only I will eat. My feet are thankful to sit down for a few moments while I type this letter. Before I digest our seven-course feast, I must first absorb and write down everything the three of us discussed in the office on Tuesday.

Thanks for your attentiveness, especially since the outlook is poor, *again!* You started by asking about my recent vacation, but I cut you short in order to get to matters at hand—my chest and armpit. Today it seems important to give you a glimpse of my Ohio.

Going home was a dream come true. I stayed in a quaint cottage on the lake where I vacationed as a child. Management (my sister) greeted me with a fire in the fireplace, oil lamps burning, chocolates, and a rose on my pillow. God knew I was comin' to town, so he arranged colorful fall foliage mixed with freshly fallen snow, elements of my two favorite seasons. What a personal welcome. You'll enjoy this: the first morning I slipped out the back door in nothing but a Floridian T-shirt and snow boots to take pictures of the golden maple tree with a frosty lake and sunrise backdrop. It was 37 degrees. Good thing the door did not lock behind me, huh? No underwear.

Over the next nine days, family members, classmates, friends, even an old band director came to visit me. Between reunions I rested and read, listened to music, shuffled through autumn leaves, ate nourishing meals, and reminisced. Communing with God, his nature, and my beloved heritage was exactly what a favorite doctor ordered.

Midweek I bought two Ohioan burial plots. Are you raising your eyebrows? You are right. Shopping for gravesites is not on America's roster of top ten vacation activities. Quite honestly, though, you must know I traveled home to say goodbye. You would too if you were suffering nagging pain in the right armpit and found a curious knot on the left ribcage, all within a short amount of time after radiation and chemotherapy. My entire torso is in turmoil. Am I walking through the valley of the shadow of death by now?

Let me go over the particulars of Tuesday's office visit. You were ninety-eight percent sure the knot on my left ribcage was malignant. I was ninety-eight percent sure the knot on my left ribcage was cancer recurring, but hearing you say it sounded worse. You cautioned me against further surgery, suggested I restart Taxotere ASAP, and somehow—two days before a holiday—you sent me right over to the imaging office for an immediate ultrasound, chest X-ray, and bone scan. Results of those scans were on your desk yesterday morning. You conferred with Dr. Cappelletti, who convinced you a needle aspiration of the rib nodule was necessary; he scheduled the procedure for *this coming Monday*, December 1! You and Cappelletti agreed to save the angry lymph nodes as treatment markers. Yesterday afternoon you [yourself] called me with scan results and the surgical appointment. Man alive! Do you and my surgeon work at lightning speed with every patient, or am I special? Thank you (I think).

Next week's pathology report will determine whether we dance or shoot up in the chemo room. Meanwhile, especially today, I will offer the sacrifice of praise to God—for life, for breath, for shelter, for loving folks, for freedom of choice, and for laughter around a table.

And I give thanks for a friend with expertise in medicine.

I pray you are in the midst of a happy, noisy crowd today. Neal and I will see you next Tuesday. Monday I meet with the funeral director at Handley's Funeral Home. (Is that more information than you asked for?)

Signed,

Connie

Connie B. Titus, a grave seeker
trying not to fear evil

Wednesday, December 10, 1997

Hello Doctor,

Pathology said I should once again shoot up some drugs in your presence, so we restarted Taxotere last week. Yesterday, were you trying to convince me Taxotere's second regimen would be less traumatic than the first, similar to labor and delivery of a second child? Well, little do *you* know. The labor/delivery of our second child was worse than the first. So go ahead, note in my chart: grumpy patient complains. We have not yet driven to the ER, for which Neal is particularly thankful, but I am being torn apart with pain.

Hey, Taxotere is a perfect name for a chemotherapy drug. It taxes you and tears you apart, one molecule at a time.

Your patient, my friend Nanette Barrish, called me last evening. The two of you discussed her poor prognosis yesterday, and she got word my future is bleak as well. For some reason, Nanette thinks I am a realistic woman with a peaceful and positive approach to death. She sounded anxious to hear my take on this hubbub of dying. The two of us compared notes about our upcoming demise. Too bad the party line is outdated. You would have loved to listen in on our conversation.

Nanette caught me off guard, yet I feebly whipped up a last-minute batch of realistic, peaceful, positive jargon, most of which I learned from you.

Pretend you are on that party line.

First off, I gently put you back into place. Physicians cannot possibly decide when or how life ends, and it is harmful to shape a patient's mind in that direction. God alone owns exclusive rights to this information. The medical staff is comprised of simple, educated, opinionated humans trained to assist and coach. God elects a good many of them. Nanette and I agreed how beautifully you shine in the coaching business. Forgive me, sir, for referring to you as simple.

Next I told a few miracle stories. People are given one year, six months, two weeks, or even an hour to live, and by some strange wonder, they are still alive today. Professionals may limit our hope to a one-percent survival rate, yet we have the right to believe we are in that one percent. The body's connection to the brain is powerful, moving us forward and/or backward.

I spoke on the topic of madness. Anger manufactures motivation for me. Personally I like the type of mad you provoke, sternly getting in my face, barking orders, etc. After I heal from the hurt, determination rushes in. I research, read, and ask a slew of questions, deciding how best to make myself comfortable, even for ten minutes at a time. Usually I fall back in love with you, but more importantly, I discover how to love and nurture myself...without you.

Nanette expressed similar mad encounters with you; however, she retreats. My friend is assertive in her teaching profession but surprisingly meek and mild as a patient, even timid when it comes to asking questions. According to Nanette, questioning the doctor is an evil practice. I tried to straighten her out. Right up to my dying days I will question you regarding dosages, reactions, alternative plans, and pain (physical and emotional) along with asking strange questions like whether or not you know how to change a fluorescent light bulb. I can then weigh your answers and run with what is useful.

You and I flourish in our love-hate relationship. I assured Nanette a love-hate relationship between survivor and the simple human in a white coat is natural and necessary. We tossed around a few ideas of how she could thrive between these two passions with you in the middle. And we laughed.

This is heartbreaking. You wrote Nanette a prescription to dance at daybreak, but she lost it and never gave it another thought. I stressed the importance. We talked ourselves through a line-dance routine over the party line. It wasn't daybreak, but what the heck.

Finally and thankfully, the cheerleading portion ended. I stepped down off the soapbox and shared Connie's stark truth. I cry every day and often find myself on the edge of complete breakdown. For a self-sufficient, independent cuss like me to give in and ask for help causes shame. I obsess over past regrets and sins. Confession and forgiveness bring little comfort. In darkness comes the fear of dying a slow, painful, wretched death and how that will affect my family.

And talk about mad! Connie Titus was ticked off twenty-four/seven last week. Mad because I felt lousy with a 0.6 white count; irritated while driving through construction in a car that stalls at stop lights; aggravated with eighty-five degree weather in winter; angry with a stupid lady in the drugstore for taking forever to count coupons and write a check for sundry items when all I needed was an emergency candy bar to get me to the clinic for blood work. Mad because life and time go on.

People have a lot of nerve, shopping with joy at Christmas. Norman Rockwell scenes make me want to vomit. Can't people see that Nanette's family and my family are suffering dreadful pain? Holidays should be cancelled and that's putting it mildly.

My mom is probably rolling over in her grave because I typed the word stupid. Little does she know I am upset and desperate enough to rip off a whole string of vulgarity—like Ralphie's father on *A Christmas Story*.[23] Did you see that movie? Remember how Ralphie's father fights with the furnace in the basement and his cursing comes up through the register with the smoke? The movie producers fixed it up cute, though; it sounds like he's cussing in a foreign language. You can't quite make out his terminology. Ha.

You can pretend your Christian friend is not capable of vulgarity or "furnace" talk, but the truth is: I am no saint.

Nanette appreciated the *I am no saint* section best of all. It's old news for Neal, and now for you.

I shared my spiritual belief that our weak moments make God so strong, so virile—and he prefers it this way. It is a new concept for Nanette. She will check it out. Despite the content of this letter, I somehow inspire Nanette in the faith department. She is teaching me the art of adventurous womanhood. On the last leg of our race, we complement each other nicely.

Are your two gals about to die? Not quite yet. Can you hang tight to the finish line? Thanks, from both of us.

Love,

Connie

Connie, a realistic, peaceful, positive madwoman who is no saint

Sunday, December 28, 1997

Dr. Collin:

My body wins. I give in. I am resigning from my dream job; from stalwart-hood; from the School of Pollyannas; from my realistic, peaceful, and positive approach; and maybe, from life itself. I surrender. No more pretending. I am sick.

All our married life I have chosen to work outside the home for the joys of purpose and contribution to family finances. Removal from the workforce is totally out of character for me. Worse yet, vacating the position with Dr. and Mrs. Morrison wounds my spirit. They offered me an opportunity of a lifetime—my debut into the medical field. This job gave me more purpose than any other, especially after my diagnosis. What a great diversion, too. I poured myself into the patients, forgetting all about my thorn, until I got into my car at day's end. Then it was as if someone pasted a big, bold banner on my windshield. "You have cancer—you could die soon!" Oh yeah, I remember.

God confuses me, granting me a meaningful job but quickly snatching it away. I gave it a good college try. I dressed in uniform and reported for work every day, even if it was only a two-hour increment. Shoot. Some days I arrived, sat down, grabbed my purse again, and drove home. Dr. Morrison invited me to do whatever, whenever. But no employer should run a business like that. They deserve a dependable, ambitious, healthy staff.

And my family deserves more. Whether I worked thirty minutes or six to eight hours, there was definitely nothing left of me for family or home life. If I can only do one thing a day, should it not be lunch with Caryn, tossing a few baseballs to Ron, or standing upright in the kitchen with a smile when Mr. Titus comes home? I think so.

Tests show my cancer has not metastasized to major

organs or bones, but in view of the fact it reared up so quickly after chemo and radiation, the outlook sucks, doesn't it? Excuse my terminology. I was in or not far from the bed for twenty days this month and fought some bad depression. No more play-acting for me. Operating like I am healthy, energetic, and whole when I am not, is exhausting. From now on I want to exercise the freedom to be weak, limp, scared, angry, or just generally messed up. Okay?

How are you? How do you cope with weak, limp, scared, angry, and generally messed up creatures all day? Do you dance at daybreak? Isn't it time for you to give us another demonstration in the chemo room? Jitterbug. Go for it, mister.

Fondly,

Connie

Connie Titus, resigned to the fact

P.S. Our church family detected my short-on-faith spirit and conducted a lovely prayer meeting for Neal, our children, and me in a friend's home a few days before Christmas. In the warmth of peaceful candlelight, folks of all ages sat Indianstyle on the floor, full circle around us, reading from God's Word and petitioning him for his healing favor. I shall never forget it. What a beautiful act of friendship.

> Is anyone sick? He should call for the elders of the church and they should pray over him and pour a little oil upon him, calling on the Lord to heal him. And their prayer, if offered in faith, will heal him, for the Lord will make him well…
>
> James 5:14-15, TLB

Friday, January 23, 1998

Dear Alan S. Collin, M.D.:

Here is an account about your buddy, Dr. Channon. But do not worry about me or him.

The depression you'll read below has not immobilized me. Obviously I am upright, moving from my bed to the computer for typing. I am not severely depressed because severe depression shows itself in lack of appetite. I have yet to miss breakfast, lunch, or dinner. I am bold enough to speak my mind. If I were truly losing ground, there would be no written record. Faint signs of a fighter show up between these lines. Please know I still consider Dr. Channon part of our team. But have a look, if you dare, where he sends me.

The specialist—he seemed like a harmless creature. His effect on me was despondency, suspension, grayness. At least this time I waited until we were in the parking lot before sobbing and wrenching. My husband sat in the driver's seat, disabled, disarmed. My lamentations killed him softly.

We still do not know what the man said to us. We sat through his lengthy dictation; he repeated himself. We still do not know what the man said to us.

I had no questions, no ideas, no interest. There seemed no reason to continue. All systems shut down.

From where I lie in my bed, I see the sky…a Bernie Siegel suggestion. During increased bedtime with disease, I see all sorts of skies—nighttime and daytime. Hues of dusk whisper either tranquility or terror. Dawn's colors are usually full of anticipation. Bright blue skies with puffy white clouds move swiftly and advertise that God is milling about up there. Storm clouds roll with the power of precipitation. Clear, crisp, starlit skies coax sweet dreams.

But this morning, as I lie motionless and stiff, the sky is gray. Not just gray, but thick gray—and oh, so still. No blue peephole through which I can reach for God's hand.

I am separated from him. The Holy Book says nothing can separate me from God's love. That is not true. A thick gray and still sky can separate me from him. I know because it is happening. I cannot find him. I am alone.

Miracles are just out of my reach. Perhaps I am not worthy after all.

I cannot mother. I cannot move myself to daily tasks. I can hardly cry.

Pain marches on. No, that's not right. Marching indicates energy and dignity. My nagging pain shuffles, but never misses a beat.

The mantel clock chimes a one-year anniversary. My personal science-fiction flick runs indefinitely. I am no better.

This is shameful behavior for a faithful, strong, Christian-like character. I just fell off my pedestal. Whom can my shattered pieces inspire now?

Apparently God hiding himself is an ancient problem. Now I am not alone with my sorrow. Solomon says, "It is the glory of God to conceal a matter…" (Proverbs 25:2, NIV). Isaiah records, "Truly you are a God who hides himself…" (Isaiah 45:15, NIV). Jeremiah talks to God, "You have veiled yourself as with a cloud so that our prayers do not reach through" (Lamentations 3:44, TLB).

I close this letter abruptly for the mantel clock chimes lunchtime. I never miss lunch.

Love,

Connie

Connie

Wednesday, January 28, 1998

Hello Trainer/Recruiter A.S.C., M.D.:

You train, recruit, direct patients through personalized regimens, hoping we get on board and choose life. That's your job. You do it well.

What is my job? Where do I fit in? What on earth am I here for? Neal says my job is stayin' alive, and he thanks me for it every day. Believe me, it is troublesome work, this self-care business, and I get awfully tired of putting so much effort into something most of the population takes for granted.

My dream job was ministering to likewise one-breasted patients within Dr. Morrison's surgical practice. But persistent disease and chemicals abolished my work ethics. I've been unemployed outside the home for one whole month now and it's a strange feeling. I bounce around with no meaning. What is my purpose, besides your Number One IBC Research Case?

Last Friday a dear spiritual mentor came to town to check on me. It was Lani's wish that we partake of a sunrise at the beach together. I gently told Lani my toxic body doesn't rock or roll at that hour. (I admit to you now, I fail miserably at daybreak dancing.) I also complained how beach outings make me grumpy. To top it off, Friday's weather forecast was lousy. She convinced me to drive her over the bridge for mist, haze, and grayness anyway. The good part is that God granted daylight and blessed our friendly encounter, even without the orange ball bursting from his ocean.

Something came over me on that misty Saturday morning drive…a strong pull of some sort. I made Neal take me back to the same beach the next day. He and I had a lovely visit there. I expressed an interest in walking by the ocean. It's funny how you continue learning new things about your longtime partner. I thought Neal hated the beach. He reminded me I was the one who had been bellyaching about Florida's environment, not him.

Neal planted me on Florida's east coast nineteen years ago and expected me to bloom. My Ohioan heart kvetched about the heat, humidity, bugs, and sand. Poor guy. For me, a family beach excursion equaled a dreaded aerobic exercise. You drag heavy coolers, lounge chairs, and bulky bags full of stuff a family might need but never use and then, just about the time you get everything set up just right, it's time to trudge back to the car with wet sand stuck to everything making it twice as heavy. And sunscreen burns the eyeballs. Does this sound relaxing or pleasurable to you? Do doctors go to the beach? Who carries your stuff?

Anyway, during Sunday's beach-awareness talk with my husband, he marked off a mile, a straight smooth path for my shaky legs between Kelsey Burgess Memorial Park and Seaside Park. Afterwards he bought me a new pair of walking shoes. I spent the last three mornings walking a mile on the boardwalk, meditating by the seashore, breathing deep the healing properties of salty sea mist. All kinds of opportunity awaits me on the island: a new grip, taking root, the power of positive thinking, setting a good example, my share of fantasy, and you'll approve of this—a new place to dance at daybreak. Are you proud of me? This Pisces finds her way home.

One year ago my consenting body stretched out on an operating table while a skillful surgeon excised a portion of my softness. I can choose to dwell on that and shiver, or I can pat myself on the back and move forward, up the shoreline, discovering purpose. I choose moving forward up the shoreline.

I just answered my earlier questions. My new job is a free-loading beachcomber. I fit in with the sea creatures. My purpose on earth is to witness and welcome each new day dawning over the Atlantic Ocean. I will live on the healing I find there. And if Earth, Wind & Fire shows up, there will definitely be dancing at daybreak.

[Excerpts from "Fantasy"]

Every thought is a dream, rushing by in a stream

bringing life to our kingdom of doing

...loving life, a new decree,

bring your mind to everlasting liberty...

And as you stay for the play

fantasy has in store for you,

a glowing light will see you through.

It's your day, shining day, all your dreams come true

as you glide, in your stride with the wind...[24]

Love,

Connie

Connie, a beachcomber, gliding
with the wind

P.S. How much longer must I take Taxotere? I do not think it
works for me anymore.

So take a new grip with your tired hands, stand firm on your shaky legs, and mark out a straight, smooth path for your feet so that those who follow you, though weak and lame, will not fall and hurt themselves, but become strong.

Hebrews 12:12-13 (TLB)

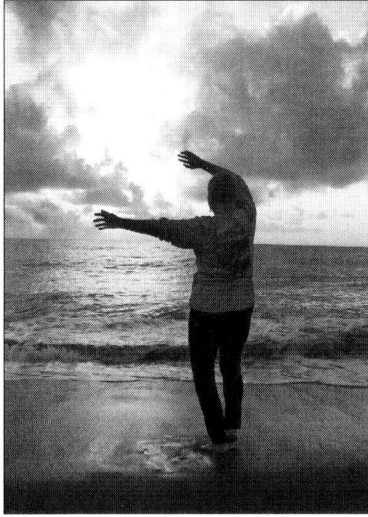

Patient Connie's new career is to welcome each new day at the ocean, raise thankful arms to heaven, and work with God at moving clouds out of the way—dancing, dancing, all the while.

Courtesy of Photographer Caryn Gonzalez

Friday, January 30, 1998

Hello Gray-Bearded Medicine Man:

I've gone haywire. Your Oncology Summit Conference on Tuesday pushed my treatment to yesterday, a Thursday, in your Holly Hill office. Wrong day, wrong office, wrong attitude. Anxiety rumbled through my body even before I ventured from bed. I should have pulled the covers over my head and stayed home.

After pleasantries in the cubicle, you and I sauntered to a not-so-familiar chemo room in search of an empty chair. You seated me and walked away. No high sign or thumbs up this go round. Never mind. I am tough. I don't need you. I have work to do.

An older gentleman sat next to me getting his first chemo. We talked, I asked questions and explained to him that I think of myself as a chemo veteran. I told him I could inspire and encourage him. But when Nurse Lison approached me with cocktail equipment I proceeded to fall completely apart—sobbing, quivering, curling up into the fetal position, as if one can comfortably do that in an extra-firm chemo chair. Yeah, I was a real inspiration for that poor old fellow. If I knew his name, I would call him and apologize. Do you know whom I am talking about? Did he come in today for his Neupogen shot?

I have never felt so alone. You and your nurses passed through the chemo room, back and forth, looking at me out of the corners of your eyes, whispering to each other, "What is the matter with Connie Titus?" But did anyone come over to hold my hand, pat me on the shoulder, inquire about my nonsense, or wink a speck of empathy my way? No. It was my first time in ten chemo treatments to behave that way, and I was all alone. Thank goodness Neal had a Holly Hill delivery to make and stopped by for a few moments. Otherwise I might have ripped out the IV and jumped through a second-story window, if you had one.

Words of advice: Strong-appearing, invincible, leader-type patients occasionally come unglued, especially if they are out of their element. They cannot hold it together all the time. When this happens, walk their way with sensitivity. Offer your hanky and/or shoulder. It's called stroking, and it only takes a moment. Please and thank you. This one attentive moment will make you the best you can be and bring a smile at day's end for both the unglued patient and you. Got it?

Even though it's my day to reprimand you, Alan S. Collin, M.D., please know I care. Put on your golden ring. "... a wise friend's timely reprimand is like a gold ring slipped on your finger" (Proverbs 25:12, MSG).

Signed,

Connie

Connie, an invincible and/or
unglued leader

P.S. In my new position as beachcomber, I will add a short "tale by the sea" to some of these letters. You are a Pisces, right? My tale might bring you pleasure. I said tale, not tail. Look below for today's addition.

• • •

Tale by the Sea

After this morning's walk, I laid my body down on the board-walk to watch cloud formations. Do you ever notice clouds are much different in the winter? Thunderheads take on majestic colors and shapes that really catch my wondrous eye. In a matter of minutes I spied an abstract star that shifted into a moose, which turned out to be an angel or a descending dove, and then spread his wings like an eagle (refusing to say what he witnessed on the other side of the globe). Before I could point them out to any bystander, my imaginative figments quickly reshaped into one cloudy question mark. My eyes closed in appreciation until I was startled by a tall, gray-bearded fellow looming over me. "Are you all right?" he inquired. He'd been working out on the adjacent boardwalk, saw me lie down, and thought I was ill, faint, or about to die. It is very nice indeed for gray-bearded men to watch over me. I should have jumped up and asked him if he wanted to dance.

A circle of cautious friends think it is not safe for me to wander the beach alone. I tell them it is safe for two reasons. Criminals don't want one-breasted women. Plus God surely will not let anything bad happen to me in the place where he heals me. My cautious friends should ask if it is safe for me to wander around Wal-mart alone. That answer would be *no!*

Wednesday, February 18, 1998

Hello? Are you there? Can you hear me now?

Is this a pattern—you on vacation at my critical times? You were gone when I suffered my first recurrence, then you were out of town when side effects of my new drug regimen sent us to the emergency room, and now I've just had the pleasure of a five-day hospitalization, without you.

This is what happened. My last Taxotere treatment hit me pretty hard. Remember? I cried through the whole thing while you and your staff strolled by, oblivious. My psyche rejected the treatment and my body responded accordingly.

Friday, February 6, Neal and our daughter, Caryn, were to scout for college housing in Gainesville. My agenda, here at home, was blood work followed by rest. Neal did not want to leave me in an ill state, so I had to practically push him out the door. I sensed I was in trouble physically before they left, but I tried not to let on. It is a Thompson tradition (Thompson is my maiden name) to pull this kind of trick while caretakers are out of town. With one stern look from me, my husband and college-aged daughter hit the road.

Eighty-year-old church friends drove me for blood work. That didn't turn out too well. My white count bottomed out at 0.6, accompanied by a fever of 101 degrees. In your absence, your partner Dr. Weisman sent us straight to the hospital. And in your absence I was going to die because Neal would kill me for pulling this Thompson trick while he was out of town.

Hospitalization is somewhat amusing. The first thing I would do with an immune-suppressed patient is stick him or her in a crowded waiting room full of flu and cold germs for two hours and fifteen minutes, wouldn't you? And when that puny one was finally assigned to a room, I would make him or her wait another four hours for any medication, even Tylenol to bring down the fever, wouldn't you? Maybe it was a test to see how high my fever could spike and how low the white count could plummet. It was my first time ever begging for a Neupogen shot, praying the drug could find at least one white cell to build upon.

Dr. Weisman assumed my care for the entire stay. Dr. Weisman, or Dr. Wise Guy, as Neal and I refer to him, is a paragraph all by himself. My observations speak out loud, but let me just ask you, "From what planet is your partner?"

Perhaps I was acting like a spoiled brat, wanting my own way, something you have witnessed many a time. But as long as I am conscious, I know my own body better than anyone, including you, and I will take an active role in making decisions. One thing led to another with your alien partner. His condescending tone worked me up into a pretty intense tizzy every day. Your prized patient Connie Titus just about plastered herself up against the fourth-story hospital window, resembling Mel Brooks on the airplane in *High Anxiety*.[25] Now aren't you sorry you couldn't enjoy that?

The finishing painful touch was talking to you in the office yesterday, a week and a half after the fact. You had no idea I was hospitalized for five days. Your alien partner failed to communicate. As far as you knew, I had come to the office for another treatment. Fat chance. What I've taken so far has not worked. Lymph nodes in my right armpit are still very much inflamed and swollen. Please get with the program, sir.

Dr. Cappelletti met with me last week. This is our plan. The lymph nodes require an open biopsy, plus there is a spot in the right breast he wants to check. Surgery is scheduled for March 23, providing my blood counts rise to the occasion. Depending on a frozen-section pathology report, while I'm still on the table, he may remove all the right lymph nodes *and* the right breast. This was radical, unexpected news. My surgeon feels the lymph node problem stems from a new primary cancer in the right breast. Cappelletti ordered another ultrasound and CT scan of the upper right chest.

In your absence, I conferred with my radiation oncologist, gynecologist, and counselor, seeking their wisdom in decision-making. Meanwhile I pursued walking or crazy disco moves at the beach followed by praying, praying, and more praying. What's the use, though? I am in the biggest mess. It is time to locate the edge of the earth and jump off.

Friends want me to see yet another oncologist at the cancer center in Port Orange. I decline. I've got what I need when you are in the room *and not on vacation.*

Forgive my cynicism. When is your next vacation, Doctor? I want to plan my trauma(s) accordingly.

After my hospital stay I baked my way to Dr. Weisman's good side and we engaged in an enlightening conversation. He knows how hard it is for cancer patients to adjust to a covering associate's personality. We laughed about our awkward interaction, and he no longer appears to be from outer space. Please know I support your R & R. If Dr. Weisman is on call and I need medical attention, I think he and I could collaborate without a hitch.

Welcome home by the way,

Connie

Connie

• • •

Tale by the Sea

As the sun rose this morning over the dark Atlantic Ocean, rays of orange light illuminated the edge of the earth. I contemplated my journey out to the jumping-off place, but a gentle voice redirected. "And if you leave God's paths and go astray, you will hear a Voice behind you say, 'No, this is the way, walk here'" (Isaiah 30:21, TLB). It seems God would rather I walk or disco along the shoreline a while longer. Good idea.

Tuesday, February 24, 1998

Dear Captain of Ships in the Harbor for Safe-Keeping:

I understand you own a home on the beach. Cool. One afternoon at the seashore, when there is no golf, no basketball, and no medical issues or emergencies, please kick back, relax, and read Robert Fulghum's amusing collection, *All I Really Need To Know, I Learned in Kindergarten.* [26] It is a high-dose injection of life. His short stories will tickle that fine-tuned funny bone of yours. You chase me around with high-dose injections, now it's my turn.

I thought of you while reading because you have tried to teach me that life is to be savored and enjoyed. Fulghum reinforces your appreciation of all the goodness surrounding us.

This is a practical book, yet funny as all get out. I laughed hard enough in places to split a gut. Neal rushed into the bedroom to check on me. He thought I was in pain.

The author has probably done, heard, seen, and felt it all. He is whimsical, eccentric, earthy, and free-spirited with such an appealing literary style. Valuable lessons pop right out, leading the reader into a nod and a smile. Now I've got a crush on Fulghum. He is another nice gray-bearded friend to assist me while I pause in life.

God wants me to learn important information while safely anchored in your harbor (chemo room) for serious repair. I am learning there is more to living than what I knew in a healthy body. I am also learning how to depend upon and trust God for daily provisions. One of Neal's mom's favorite sayings is: "The Lord will provide!" That he does.

And now, Connie Titus "leaps into faith much as she earlier leaped into trouble."[27]

One of these days, with Jehovah's help, you and I will probably patch up this vessel of mine so I can sail the high seas again. All the good tidbits you and Fulghum teach me will be living freight for the destination. I am grateful.

Signed,

Connie

• • •

Tale by the Sea

One lone sailboat sat offshore in this morning's foggy mist— one lone captain of one lone ship. I thought I saw you, *El Capitan*. Did you have the day off?

Sunday, March 22, 1998

Dr. Collin,

It's me.

Well, tomorrow are the biopsies. Two cuts: right breast and right axilla. This is the sixth time Dr. Cappelletti has chased me down the hallway with his knife. You would think he and I could find something better to do.

I am joking on the outside, dreading the ordeal on the inside. If pathology proves positive, it will be the fourth malignancy in fifteen months despite two different chemo regimens, high-dose radiation, and multiple surgeries. Experts seem concerned. My situation cannot be promising.

Is now a good time to talk about death? You have silenced me several times. Is that your stance, we should never talk of death?

Hear ye, hear ye—untried resources of a one-breasted brain.

My eldest sister sent me an article on MIA doctors—doctors who go missing in action when their patients are about to die. Even with patients they have treated for years, doctors go MIA to avoid saying goodbye, leaving their patients perplexed and abandoned in their vulnerable state. The old medical school teaches the thought that if a patient dies, the physician has somehow failed. And some doctors are afraid to show emotion, thinking it an unprofessional behavior. But are these justifiable reasons to go missing in action? Poppycock.

The article suggests physicians should step up to the plate and tell their dying patients how their time together has contributed to the doctor's learning experience and ability to better care for patients in the future. Terminal patients, at the end of life, want an opportunity to say thank you to the doctor. They want that moment to reassure, "I don't think this is a failure. I appreciate what you've done for me."

Dr. Collin, don't be a doctor missing in action. I, for one, would want to express my grateful heart, and I also would be incredibly touched that you cared enough to be teary-eyed. Honest, human emotion shared between two trustworthy friends at this point can only be a gift.

If you have trouble with death talk, maybe you should take up practice in the UK. Instead of the word death, they use the terminology *negative patient outcome*. Isn't that funny? Call it whatever you like, put aside your fears and let us deal with my needs, please. Come on, Doc. I will be gentle.

Walking daily with a terminal illness forced me into an ongoing conversation with my Creator. He was waiting patiently for me. When I approached his bench, he seemed quite familiar with my name and predicament. Many family members and friends are bugging God with prayer on my behalf. Moses was able to change God's mind with prayer. God hears and heeds the petitions of those who love him. I realize our Father's way of answering prayer may be very different from what we have in mind. And let's face it. We are all going to die of a cause. Persistent IBC is most likely going to be my cause. Or then again, maybe I'll step off the curb tomorrow and be run over by a celery truck.

My biggest fear is dying a slow, drawn-out kind of death, with a lot of mess and misery. I read terrifying stories on the Inflammatory Breast Carcinoma support group website. One woman bled from her eyes, ears, nose, mouth, etc. Neal curtailed my IBC support group involvement after showing him these stories. IBC is an aggressive strain, and it usually takes you downhill fast. Fast is a plus, though, in this respect.

Bold in prayer, I placed my order with God and gave him three choices as to how I shall depart from this earth. I would not mind dropping dead on the boardwalk, keeling over on the altar steps in our church after singing a rousing choral anthem, or hearing someone say, "Oh, my God! She's dead? I just saw her in the produce department at Publix this morning!"

Neal doesn't want me to die without him by my side. He thinks we could have some of our most tender, intimate moments at that time. Maybe he's right. But I'm not sure I can bear the loneliness in his eyes. I'd rather sneak out while Neal's not looking or when he is sleeping. Our local radio station plays Frank Sinatra singing "Softly" all the time lately. Frank makes me cry.

> Softly, I will leave you softly, for my heart would break, if you should wake, and see me go. So I leave you softly, long before you miss me, long before your arms can beg me stay, for one more hour, or one more day. After all the years, I can't bear the tears to fall, so softly I leave you there.[28]

I am in the midst of heaven research. Drawing from Scripture and what the old folks talk about and also from the wisdom of little children, this is my understanding of death, dying, and heaven thus far:

1. If we love the Lord and trust him, we take our last breath here on earth and our first breath in heaven with him. (Read 2 Corinthians 5:6, TLB)

2. He has prepared for us a mansion with many rooms and there we will live forevermore, in our new bodies. (Read John 14:2, NIV; 2 Corinthians 5:1, NIV)

3. I believe we will be greeted by and reunited with our loved ones who have already passed. Perhaps they give us the guided tour, or maybe it's Jesus himself.

4. Our eternal home must be gorgeous—full of brilliant light and glory, clarity, color, purity, and gems, which translate to me as complete peace, laughter, love, and dancing. I see endless dancing on the streets of gold. (Read Revelation 21:10-27, NIV)

5. Harp music? Hmm. I am not sure about harp music. I am more a Dixieland, Jazz, or Pop Rock gal. Hopefully the Lord will usher me into the right concert hall.

6. There is no pain, disease, loneliness, abuse, sadness, homesickness, or tears in heaven. (Read Revelation 21:4, TLB)

7. Those experiencing near death see the lovely possibilities of this eternal home and decide right there and then they don't want to go back to earth.

8. No one is married in heaven. We are one big happy family of angels. (Read Matthew 22:30, TLB)

9. Yes, there will be a kind of judgment process near the Pearly Gates to find out in which department we will be stationed, but this isn't as bad as it sounds because our Lord is full of grace, mercy, and love abundant. (Read 2 Corinthians 5:10, TLB)

10. In the language of babes, "I think heaven would have fences in it with strawberries. David who fighted Goliath would be there, too. I think heaven would have blueberries and gold in it. Old people will be there and God's angels. There also will be a big, big feast that keeps everybody full." Andrew Edwards, age three.

Does my belief and trust prevent me from shaking in my shoes at sundown? The answer is no. I am human. Death and dying is still a journey to the unknown. But if I spend time focusing on the above researched promises, I have a better chance to pull this voyage off with joy. Yes, Dr. Collin, I said joy!

Now, can I tell you something weird, as if the first forty letters are normal? Twice last week I heard familiar voices in my sleep calling my name. I woke up thinking someone was beckoning me to come hither. One more thing…after you read this, you will ask your staff to reserve my room at the local loony bin…I smell cigarette smoke. For three-to-four-day spans, I constantly smell cigarette smoke in my house, in my car, in the choir loft, in Publix. Wherever I go, a cloud of cigarette smoke follows me. No one else smells it. No one in our family smokes. No visitors are allowed to smoke in or around our property. I do not frequent bars or smoky restaurants where smoke becomes imbedded in nose hair. My daddy used to smoke Camels. Not lately, though. He's been dead for years. Could his spirit be near me during these episodes?

Are you shaking your head? Remember, I am a research project. Folks from every faith come into your office. Diverse outlooks must be interesting. Thank you for hearing me out.

I might be jumping the gun with death talk since pathology won't be on your desk until week's end. Wouldn't that be a pleasant surprise? I'll see you Tuesday, March 31, for either a celebration dance or a new plan of action.

Love,

Connie

Connie, your gal with a possible negative patient outcome

• • •

Tale by the Sea

In the midst of such a magnificent landscape, our Creator bids me to be still and know him. "Do you want more and more of God's kindness and peace? Then learn to know him better and better" (2 Peter 1:2, TLB). There is no finer place to know him better and better than at my beach.

April Fool's Day, 1998

Alan S. Collin, M.D.:

The vote is in, not in my favor. I am now working my way to negative patient outcome. This is no April Fool's joke.

Last Friday, Dr. Cappelletti's nurse pulled, and pulled, and pulled ten yards of drainpipe out of my side while Cappelletti paced the floor reading the pathology report, to which he tacked on a personal, "I am sorry." He described my right armpit as a matted mass. My learned surgeon still claims it must be a new primary malignancy stemming from the right breast, yet he could not find the breast lesion he went in to biopsy. Reports confirm that Inflammatory Carcinoma traveled across the sternum, skipped the right breast, and nestled into the right armpit. No trail in sight. This is unheard of except in the body of Connie Titus. Eight of twenty lymph nodes excised from the right axilla were malignant. Tally now, from both armpits, a total of twenty-one lymph nodes positive with cancerous tumors. Am I the first who lives to tell this story?

Yesterday, the pain on your face as you looked at the pain on our faces strangely softened the agony. We met for one of those muted office visits where nothing productive took place, and I thank you. Thank you for not pressing us with plans or decisions. God knows how I hate decisions, plus I am not capable at this moment. Were any words spoken? You, Neal, and I sat rather motionless wondering which direction to go. Aggressive chemotherapy drugs, consolidated radiation therapy, and surgical removal with clean margins cannot shut down this disease. It wants me.

I came away from the appointment realizing options are few to none. No sleeping last night. My friend J. Ellsworth Kalas says when I receive a message that upsets me, I should seek the Lord penitently rather than resenting the messenger.[29] I do not resent you, Dr. Collin, but I did consult with the Lord in my restlessness. His response was "...choose life...love the Lord your God, listen to his voice, and hold fast to him" (Deuteronomy 30:19-20, NIV). That sounds easy...for one with strong faith. I have not made the grade yet.

Yesterday ended and today began with a remembrance. Early on someone suggested that I look under every rock for a cure. I did not know what their statement meant, nor did I care. I assumed they were referring to alternative, complimentary rubbish like colon cleansing or drinking carrot juice until your hands turn orange. Conventional Connie wanted no part of it. Besides, I have you and trust you for all the answers. Negative patient outcome can change values pretty quickly, though. Today I am ready to look under every rock or even grab short straws.

Between now and our next visit April 14, I will visit health-food stores, consult with the nutritionist in your Holly Hill Cancer Clinic, and schedule appointments with a Chinese herbalist, homeopathic doctor, and massage therapist. I want to read and research everything I can get my hands on regarding wellness and implement my own natural program. Do not worry. Moderation is my key. No coffee enemas or orange hands for me.

You are still co-chairman of my body. Help me grab straws and look under every rock. I will bring my alternative sketch soon. At that time, please greet me with your best open mind.

Until then,

Connie

Connie, striving for positive patient outcome

Tale by the Sea

The surgery site hurts like the dickens, so about the best I can do dance-wise at Seaside Park is the Hokey-Pokey. And I'm choosy about what I put in and shake all about. I do know peace can be found over the bridge and through the sea grass. No coolers or lounge chairs are necessary. No family or friends. It is simply me, a pair of dance shoes, Blues Brothers' sunglasses covering bloodshot tears, a straw hat, a bottle of pure water, and a feeble prayer on my lips, asking, "Is anything too hard for God?" (Genesis 18:14, TLB). Before you ponder if there are any articles of clothing between the dance shoes and Blues Brothers' glasses, yes, my body is covered, at least the top part. Your pondering tickles me into a blush, though, so thank you.

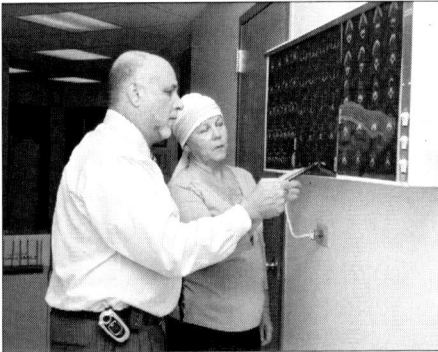

Dr. Collin and Patient Connie investigate CT scan films showing third recurrence and discuss why her liver looks like a manatee.

Courtesy of Photographer Jerry Brewer

Wednesday, April 15, 1998

Dear Dr. Collin:

We have been working on this thing for a while. Each office visit explores a step, an emotion. I take something profound you say to me, and either chuckle, bristle, shed a hurtful tear, or mount up with wings and fly. Oh, yeah. I can roll my eyes as good as you can.

First let me tell you: Neal and I both appreciate your agreeable attitude yesterday. You were so agreeable, there must be a misunderstanding. Are you okay? Are you running a fever?

During my hospitalization in February I decided against any more aggressive treatment methods. It's just not me. While delivering that well-rehearsed speech, you threw a curve ball, agreeing with me, of all things! I was dumbfounded for the duration. I completely lost my balance and couldn't make heads or tails out of what followed. Wonders never cease. This is one visit I should have recorded.

I do remember discussing numbers—low numbers and response rates to Arimidex, a tiny white pill that should not help any ER/PR negative gal. I made a face. Then, I believe the next thing you said to me, in your best gentle, lecture voice was, "We will see progression with this. I don't know when, or how, or to what degree, but we will make and see progress. I'm sure of it."

At the time and for hours later, your statement sounded like a warming, strength-building spiritual cheer to me, for me, until later that evening when I talked to my eldest sister, Jerry, who asked, "Was your doctor referring to a healing or the cancer?"

Oh, my God, no. Did you mean the cancer would progress? No, no, you meant conquering the beast, controlling it, beating it didn't you? Did you say *make progress* or *see prog-*

ress? Was the term *progress* or *progression?* Oh, God. I don't know. Dr. Collin, I thought you were assuring me my cup is half-full.

I felt an overwhelming need to call you first thing this morning to find out just what you meant.

Well, I won't call, I won't ask. We are leaving for a family outing this weekend to Gainesville and Old Town in Kissimmee. I choose to remain with my first instinct. It gives me unlimited hope, and my body responds to optimistic mindsets. Neal does not remember you saying any of this, so he is no help. Perhaps you don't remember either. Whatever was said and whatever my connotation, be assured that I still own a healthy attitude on the subject of death. Mr. Titus and I do not have our heads in the sand. My days have already been numbered and recorded by my loving Father. We are driving to Gainesville. I can watch for hospital signs along the highway or I can put my life in God's capable hands, trusting him to work through this man-doctor named Alan S. Collin, M.D. Cure or no cure.

For the first time in my life, I am really living. In the midst of pain, fear, hard work, and confusing statements from the doctor, exhilaration sneaks in.

Thanks, friend, for hope, even if it was a misunderstanding.

With appreciation,

Connie

Connie

P.S. Neal filled the Arimidex prescription on the way home yesterday and I took my first dose this morning. I pray it works well with the vitamins and supplements lined up on my kitchen counter.

Tale by the Sea

I try to dance barefoot in the surf's early morning beauty at least three or four times a week. The surge of refreshment is well worth driving twenty-two miles round trip. I don't care who sees me or what they think. And I don't always need music. Once that first wave hits my big toe, I am plugged into the current and rhythm of the Creator of our universe. God's abundant love floods my soul with beautiful music. Day by day I dig my feet (not my head) deeper into the wet sand where God and my husband planted me. "May your roots go down deep into the soil of God's marvelous love…" (Ephesians 3:17, TLB).

Sunday, May 3, 1998

You in the White Coat!

Tuesday's appointment went fairly well, yes? You looked over and accepted my alternative plan with grace. I am impressed. Most medical doctors hate that kind of stuff. Are you still trying to decipher my list of questions? Thank you for remaining calm when I pound you with tough concerns. Dilemmas over what to do next are very tiring for both of us.

Cancer patients are locked into a perpetual decision-making process. Technical choices of surgery, drugs, radiation, etc., are not as important as emotional choices such as mindset, disposition, or visions. I am on a roll trying to make emotional choices and need your help.

Will fear, pain, and humility consume me, or will I hike ahead with a Divine escort? Shall I rise and dance in the morning or stay in bed staring blankly at cobwebs behind the curtains? Do I ask questions or shuffle into your office accepting every shot and injection—like you are King of the World and I have no opinion? What's my capacity to roll with the punches?

I just asked for your help but decided to talk it over with my Lord instead. From his ever-ready, ever-willing heart, he gives wisdom. "If you want to know what God wants you to do, ask him, and he will gladly tell you, for he is always ready to give a bountiful supply of wisdom to all who ask him; he will not resent it" (James 1:5, TLB).

Wisdom for my choice-making looks like this:

Fear of death, physical suffering, and an unrecognizable body are enough to shove me over the edge just about every morning of the week. Admitting my desperation and writing it down gives me the ability to steer away from the edge, though, and move about under the umbrella of God's compassionate attention.

I give permission for a few listless *oh, woe is me* days, and you read them all. Afterwards my human feet are then anxious to dance sometime between sunrise and sunset. And despite recent horrid news, there is still Vintage Wine lipstick, earrings, and drawn-on eyebrows even for the beach (especially for the beach). I aim for womanhood.

We've all read about taking charge of our own healthcare. What a wise and powerful cue. I crave information from celebrated professionals and own nearly a complete library of books, tapes, and pamphlets on this subject. Someone gave me a little notebook to keep my running list of questions and observations. You probably dread the sight of it. With research and my little notebook, I am able to take control and maneuver you somewhat, oh ye respected and honorable king.

About a patient's running list of questions/observations: is it a prerequisite of your partnership to snatch everyone's list from their hand the moment they enter an exam room? You do it to me, and I've heard your associates do it to their patients. I even watched you grab a list from Nanette in the hospital one day, but it was Clancy's list of items to bring from the house. Remember the third item? "Underwear—no thongs!" Tee hee—a hospital room full of blushing professionals. From that point on, I decided to write all my lists in code. It can be your crossword puzzle.

• • •

Patient Connie's code list from Tuesday's visit is so efficiently coded, Patient cannot decipher.

• • •

Am I choosing to turn the other cheek with four malignancies in fifteen months? Definitely. Certain activities boost the immune system and encourage me to forget harsh numbers. I start by attending early dawn by the sea and, although I'm no ballerina, God enjoys my honest efforts. When the Titus Family Band gathers, I at least hold an instrument near my lips. I harmonize in the choir loft. Seeds have been planted. Weeds are ripped right out of the ground and toted to the pasture *by me.* The healing power of laughter stimulates a sound response to life. You taught me all you know about that subject. Angels inside ordinary people show up on my doorstep and do their thing. A total body massage followed by Heath Bar Frozen Yogurt causes me to sigh with pleasure. I occasionally resort to temper tantrums while wearing chicken slippers, which proves "there are seasons of the human soul. The warrior of one day can be the frightened child of another."[30]

Attached is a copy of my natural alternative plan. Bind it in my chart, please. You slay me. While reading down through the activity list, you questioned the placement of sex. Where do you want me to put sex—between worship and Bible study, or next to family dinners?

Next Tuesday, let's have some fun, you and me. I'll demonstrate my latest dance step, you follow my instruction. Chemo patients will love it. I will wear chicken slippers. You wear argyle socks. It will be a Hay Day, for sure.

Love from a sassy/scared friend,

Connie

Connie

Connie's Alternative Plan for Healing
Beginning April 1998

Herbal Tonic: (Daily)

Floressence (turkey rhubarb, burdock, slippery elm, sheep sorrel, kelp, red clover blossom, milk thistle) 1-2 oz. mixed with equal amount of distilled water, one hour before breakfast.

Supplements: (Daily)

Vitamins A, B-50, C, E, Caltrate D, Flaxseed Oil, Evening Primrose Oil, one aspirin.

Other Nutritional Agents: (Daily)

Crystalized ginger; green tea; Echinacea spray; seven whole almonds; soy shakes; eight 8 oz.-glasses of distilled water; foods from the antioxidant/anti-cancer list below.

Antioxidants

Apples, bananas, beets, broccoli, Brussels sprouts, corn, garlic, pink grapefruit, kale, kiwi, oranges, plums, red grapes, red peppers, spinach, and tea.

Anti-Cancer Grocery List

I don't know if there is any truth to this, but I load up my cart with: almonds, apples, apricots, barley, beets, broccoli, Brussels sprouts, cabbage, carrots, cauliflower, celery, chickpeas, corn, cucumbers, figs, flax seed, garlic, ginger, grapes/raisins, greens, herbs, horseradish, lentils, nuts/seeds, oats, onion, orange peel, parsley, pineapple, potatoes, radishes, rhubarb, rice, rutabaga, rye, soybeans, spinach, sprouts, squash, strawberries, sunflower seeds, sweet potatoes, tea, tomatoes, turnips, watercress, wheat, wild mushrooms, and yogurt. *This is an incomplete list. I did not include items I dislike or have no idea what they are.

Activities (in no particular order):

Beach; deep breathing salty sea mist; walking; sex; monthly massage; worship; Bible study; singing; dancing; brass duets with my hubby; pulling weeds; planting seeds; fifteen minutes of sunshine; writing; visitation; photography; traveling to Bellefontaine, Ohio, in the autumn, and Roslyn, Washington, in the wintertime; old movies; Northern Exposure and Bill Cosby; cleaning closets; Glad and Alvin Slaughter and Azuza Pacific University Choir; family dinners; tobogganing; skydiving; the Tiki Bar on a Saturday evening; and Earth, Wind & Fire.

Saturday, May 16, 1998

Sir:

Was I wasting your time? You called me in, remember? I was perfectly content between my Martha Stewart sheets. Sick, but content.

I apologize ahead of time for the content of this letter. Connie Titus has been known to sugar-coat, but you will not see it here. If I thought it, wrestled with it, or blew it out of proportion, it's in this letter. No pussyfooting. Got it? Now read on, exercising caution.

Is there a pattern on my sick/sad days? In my opinion, we might work out a better system. Let me refresh your memory. Thursday morning I drove to your Ormond-By-The-Sea office for a regular check up. You were happy to see my face tan, my body agile, and my spirits high. We agreed to continue the current treatment plan of Arimidex. As usual, you offered sufficient time and support. I left you for my dance on the beach—the samba.

A Brazilian dance must not agree with a German/English gal because I felt lousy all of a sudden. It worsened as the day went on, and I ended up shaking with chills Thursday night. I notified your office yesterday morning. You called me in for a chest X-ray and battery of cultures.

Unlike the day before, my face was red and swollen from crying, my body clammy with fever, and my spirits, well, I won't print that here. After your detached poking and prodding, and reporting you saw nothing at all inside my head, I lay alone for an hour or more on a hard table, waiting, waiting for cultures and X-rays to be conducted and read.

You finally waltzed my way and, with your back towards me, rattled off results and instructions so fast, I could not understand a word you said. Being foggy with fever cuts any brain function. You gruffly motioned me toward the checkout desk. Walking swiftly ahead, you muttered a comment to Nurse Nicole, slapped my chart on the counter, handed me four prescriptions, and then passed me like some ship in the night. No "Sorry you are hurting," or "Let me know how you are doing." Not even a bloody goodbye.

Why don't you just stab me in the heart with one of Cappelletti's knives?

I was so freakin' mad. I called Neal and told him that when it is time for me to die he is to keep you away from me. I don't want you making me sad or mad on my deathbed. Except we think I live longer than average IBCers because of certain mad spells with you. Is this your ultimate goal today, increasing my life expectancy with gruff detachment?

Stuff the gruff detachment. Let this be sufficient notice: When I crawl towards the finish line, you are to sit on the edge of my bed, look into my eyes, and for God's sake, say something sweet. A kiss on the forehead wouldn't hurt either.

You and I have engaged in conversations about your practice evolving through the years. In your late twenties, early thirties, you strictly treated the disease. You and your patients worked against each other, dry and agitated. There were no relationships. You just about threw in the towel. I'm not certain who shed light or what changed, but between the ages of mid-thirty and mid-forty, you discovered how to nurture a whole person.

You and your patients thrive in each other's company now, except for me on sick/sad days. When I need compassion, empathy, or a few extra minutes the most, you either bark a lecture or act like I'm bothering you. Why?

As early as last night, I softened. I made excuses for you.

Could it be you hurt when I hurt and you don't know how to express it? Maybe you don't want to coddle, afraid I might become weak and pull the sheet up over my head. Perhaps you refuse to lead me adrift with compassion, lest I cling too tight. Or you could simply be frustrated by office hours never flowing; demands piling up, smothering you; or the way death, for some, is imminent, despite your concentrated efforts and this...stabs you...like a knife. Or tee-off time is 1:00 p.m. and this wimpy crowd had better clear out!

Whatever. Next office visit I will appear in a business-like suit with a clear head. I will stand while you sit. In fact, you can put on one of those blue paper gowns, and I will lay you down on the table for cross-examination. I will conduct your appointment, bark instructions, and slap your chart on the front counter.

Again, I'm thinking of some kind of communication device. How about flashcards? Flashcards would indicate exactly what I need from you, when, and to what degree. But the interaction would not be genuine, I suppose. Oh, well, flashcards stay at home. I'll take my chances on a genuine doctor-patient interaction, being what it may.

Connie

. . .

Tale by the Sea

The beach beckoned me to come this morning, even though it was misty and gray. No samba today. I sauntered. Salty sea mist and the tide's rush untwisted my warped thinking enough to come 'round right in this letter to you. God certainly shows himself there. He urged me to forgive you.

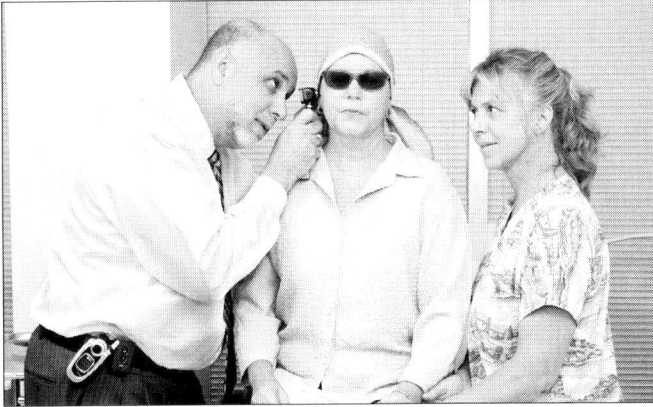

Patient is invisible when she wears dark glasses. Dr. Collin and Nurse Nicole confirm what Husband Neal has known all along. Patient Connie's brain matter is missing. Anyone can see right through her. Behold the invisible and sheer Patient Connie.

Courtesy of Photographer Jerry Brewer

Thursday, May 28, 1998

Good Morning!

I gotta tell you. I am in love with my life. Sound funny? Untimely? Do I still have cancer, or what? Is my head screwed on tight?

Yes, I probably still have cancer. And yes, my head looks level in the mirror, with hair I might add.

An unseen friend motivates me to scramble from the cancer pits toward mountain peaks, of which there are many. The exhilaration I find on the mountain peak acts as a shield on the way down again. I am happy with this course. I love marching up and down the mountains with my thoughts, all of them—even the nasty, ugly ones. At least I am alive to express them.

Yes, I still cry, fight physical pain, and wonder how serious my disease is. Obsessive grievance over body alterations continues. I think about death, hoping it is later rather than sooner. But if it takes place at 4:00 this afternoon, my family and I will be well taken care of by a gentle God. It is by his good grace I move out of the pit to busy myself, laugh a little, savor food and people, and breathe in salty sea mist while I follow your foolish dance prescription. Oh, and get this: I find myself making future plans. How strange is that? Are survivors with poor prognoses allowed to project? Well, it is partly your doing, Professor. You instruct us accordingly. What grade do I earn today?

People say I am a picture of health, a young woman with a bright and shining future in a blue swimsuit that's flat on one side. I am beginning to believe it.

Doctor, does this letter make sense? You know, I still wonder if you read these letters. I pray so. At least those that are upbeat.

Love from the center of who I am,

Connie

Connie

Tale by the Sea

This morning I walked myself into a good sweat, stripped to that flat, blue bathing suit, danced an Irish jig as best a German/English gal can, and waded out chest-deep into the cool, understanding sea. This is the nicest thing I could do for myself. The whole ocean belonged to me. There my Father, the Potter, shaped me for the rest of the day: weightless, burden-free, buoyant, and best of all, painless, in his salt water. I am not sure if the Potter shapes me for noble purpose or common use. "Does not the potter have the right to make out of the same lump of clay some pottery for noble purposes and some for common use?" (Romans 9:21, NIV).

Friday, June 12, 1998

Dr. C.:

Whew! Tuesday was another constructive office visit for me.

I walked around with my emotional antenna stuck in the "up" position, for a month…lots of rumination going on.

You just cleared my head.

I've got it now.

I am settled.

Thank you.

Bless you for dealing kindly with all the emotional antenna people who frequent your office.

I spied a greeting card with your name on it the other day. On the front cover was a short, young man, possibly age five, dressed in a sports jacket, dress slacks, and a top hat that was way too big for him. Oh, and red shoes. He was playing the fiddle.

This little musician created a soothing image of you. While you circulate among examining and hospital rooms listening to all the woe, strife, and rumination, you must be tempted to play the fiddle or your bassoon. Go ahead. I love the idea. Acoustics in the hospital corridor must be musically pleasing. Patients and staff would get such a kick out of you, especially if you wear a top hat that is way too big for you. Call me. I'll come do some kind of interpretive dance. We can be a one-man, one-woman traveling show.

God gives us talents and gifts, and we most definitely should use them. Neal's not sure I possess any talent in the dance department, but you ordered it, so I try.

"Now there are varieties of gifts, but the same Spirit; and there are varieties of services, but the same Lord; and there are varieties of activities, but it is the same God who activates all of them in everyone" (1 Corinthians 12:4-6, NRSV).

Thanks, too, for doubling as English Professor. My vocabulary increases in your care. I've been a ruminator since childhood but never knew it.

Connie

Sunday, September 6, 1998

Hi, Dr. Collin:

Here is a topic I bet most lopsided patients never discuss with any doctor.

Take a pendant, put it on a long chain (or short chain for that matter), and hang it around a mastectomy patient's neck. See what happens when she moves about.

The necklace will not hang down the center. It sways over to the empty side. If I am without prosthesis and sweating, the pendant or charm swings immediately to the void and plasters itself there. If I wear my fake booby inside a pocketed bra creating a perfect balance, jewelry still hangs crooked. Always.

You simply see a scar on my chest. I see a flattened left chest wall exposing the heart and its rhythm. Frankly, in my opinion, my heart and its rhythm are scarred. Whatever the real case scenario, I prefer to wear spiritual symbols of some sort—a pendant, locket, or charm representing the love of God. While walking on the beach today, a golden angel swung over and stuck to the scar over my heart.

What do you think this swinging pendulum phenomenon means?

I believe it means God is aware of my void and the grief that comes with it, so he swings an angel or another symbol over to protect my heartbeat. I believe it means my Creator is alive and well, and since I've been taught that his banner over me is love, I stretch my imagination and can see him actually placing that banner of love straight onto my scar line. And there it sticks.

I keep adding charms to my chain thinking the weight will surely pull it down straight. Nope. No deal. Everything swings to the left. My favorite three charms are a cross, a gift from my church family; a dancing Colorado tree, a gift from my friend in Dr. Cappelletti's office; and a cameo angel, a token of my husband's love. These three charms dance and jingle together on top of my scarred heart.

Doctor, you've noticed and commented on my cross before. Is that because it hangs crooked, or do you consider its meaning? I consider its meaning too. But for right now, I'm just glad it sticks to me.

Signed,

Connie

Connie, with sticky charms

P.S. Six-month scans are scheduled for Wednesday, October 7. We'll get together for the results on the following Tuesday, but I can tell you right now, there is no more cancer problem. Arimidex, the drug that isn't supposed to help me one bit, is helping me two bits, four bits, six bits, a dollar.

November, 1998

Alan S. Collin, M.D.:

Our office appointment of October 13 makes this upcoming Thanksgiving season a whopper for me. Can you believe it? Connie Titus is cancer free! I hope you are happy, too.

Greeting cards and letters are making your citrus box quite heavy, but I must not let a holiday slip by without awarding you another star—especially Thanksgiving, your favorite holiday. Are you headed for your quiet, colorful oasis in the mountains? I pray God will grant you refreshment wherever.

And now for your written star: Every day is Thanksgiving Day when a cancer patient can rise in the morning and say, "I feel good today. I think I will run here or there." But before our feet start running the race, or dancing the dance, it is a good and proper thing for us to bow on bended knee and give thanks to our Creator for his constant abiding love and also for sending us extraordinary people who physically guide us. That would be you, for one. Even on mad, sad, or sick days, despite what I have written on previous pages, I can honestly say I am pleased you are my doctor and teacher. You coach me with cute suggestions, examples, and pictures.

The other day I noticed you wearing running shoes. That's a new look for you. I pictured you running from the clinic, flailing your arms, when cancerous brains go off on tangents. Cute suggestive pictures of you are worth more than a thousand words. They boost white cells.

Thanks too for encouraging my gift of writing. Every now and then I consider taking frank thoughts and rumination to print. If I can inspire just one other person, it would be a worthy project.

One more thing: When it comes time for you to retire, relocate, or take a leave of absence, be reminded—I need at least one year's notice. Refer to the fine-print clause in our Doctor-Patient Contract.

Seven months into Arimidex, I experience minimal side effects, but today I don't give them any mind. I walk away from the computer, stretching and prepping for today's dance on the boardwalk. Neal and I will see you when you get back from giving thanks. You can then schedule those scans you seem to think I need.

Connie

. . .

Tale by the Sea

When I walk or dance under the shelters of the long boardwalk, the temperature is at least ten degrees cooler and breezy. Sometimes my hat flies off. Thank God I've got hair now. You should have seen children and adults' shock, watching a pudgy, middle-aged bald woman dance to no music.

Tuesday, December 15, 1998

No salutation today.

Did you receive my Thanksgiving greeting? Do you recognize my adoration and the honor it brings? Good. That was a month ago. Right now I could punch you unconscious. You are about to experience a woman converting from a delicate flower into an untamed shrew. I am stomping through the house with my chicken slippers on, shooting fire from my eyeballs and nostrils, muttering *your* name. Watch out. The pages you hold might self-destruct.

How many times, since all this started, have I called your office in desperation? The answer is once. Yesterday I left two messages. You never called back. Not one single soul from a three-office operation bothered to call. I don't care how busy your Holly Hill Monday is. I am a paying patient, too—a sick paying patient.

For nine days I've been lying around with a chest cold. The Cipro you prescribed did nothing. Although my temperature is normal, I cough so much my throat is raw. Deep breathing reveals a rattle. My voice is hoarse. The cough is dry and unproductive. I am weak, listless, and completely miserable with no patience. My church needs me to do some serious singing this weekend and they want to know what you are going to do about my condition. So I put in a call.

Another reason for my desperate call was worry over my friend Nanette Barrish. She learned the other day her tumor markers are sky high. Today she starts a new treatment with you. Nanette and I have been in a neck-to-neck race, competing to see who gets to go *home* first...but neither wants to win. This is hard, when one falls behind and one goes ahead. Even though I'm probably sicker than she is right now, I am the one going ahead...with survivor's guilt. Yet I don't want you to give me a bad cancer report to even the score.

Back to my anger: So you couldn't pick up the lousy phone and call me. And I fell through the cracks with your staff. What happened to the days when doctors made house calls?

All day yesterday, into the night, and even today, the hurt stings, anger boils.

Here we go again. Why is it…when I am really needy… you jump overboard, are unreachable, or on vacation? Don't I measure up since my cancer is on a stable level right now? Am I invisible? If I had two breasts, would you see to my concerns? I owe you money and possibly my insurance is of lower grade. Do these financial issues knock me into the *don't bother* category? If I played or talked golf, would you be more attentive?

I know. You are way too busy, stretched like Saran wrap around dozens of critical cases. What does this mean? This is my third winter under your care. I am fully aware of your hectic agenda with snowbirds and local patients on deathbeds day in and day out. So, what does this mean? Moderately sick cancer survivors should call a general practitioner or 911? At least your nurse or office gal could inform me thus.

This sucks, buddy. I am mad. On a positive side, here again, mad seems to add months, maybe years to my life span. In fact, Neal encourages me to get mad with Alan S. Collin as much and as often as possible. At least it gets him off the sharp hook. I also do some of my best writing while angry. Ruffled feathers can be a plus.

But seriously, this indifference scares me, especially as I project into the future. When it comes time for me to die, will you return my phone call? I need you, for Christ's sake! What am I doing? Ending a paragraph with reference to Christ in a letter to a Jewish man?

This Christ of mine (and my husband) inform me I am selfish; I should give poor Dr. Collin a break and get a grip on reality. They remind me I am only suffering a cold and a little emotion.

Okay. I admit it. I am sick and medicated, which makes me irrational. I am probably PMSing, even though you confirmed menopause with a blood test nine months ago. Chances are if I approached you in this condition, you would label me depressed—a doctor's catch-all statement and an observation loaded with testosterone. I am not depressed, mister-know-it-all. Depression involves days, weeks, months on end of insomnia, lethargy, loss of appetite. I never miss a meal, remember? It's plain old anger. And this too shall pass.

I question the motive behind my intense emotion and sometimes I hide from God. This morning, though, he caught up with me. We had a frank discussion about this very thing. I ranted and raved. He listened with empathy. The Lord knows my innermost thoughts of you.

Like many female cancer patients, I have fallen a little bit in love with my male oncologist. Office visits are frequent. The prognosis is followed by complicated treatment, with significant support. There is an unspoken yoke between us. You are the chief navigator in my journey to recovery. I need you. A little bit of love is a normal, natural response.

When you waltz into the examining room, I see a humorous, fascinating, sensitive and physically attractive man, although sensitive is under investigation as I speak. All right, I confess. I have, on occasion, entertained the notion of sleeping with you. (Cancer patients are allowed fantasies too, right?) Don't get nervous. You and I will not remake the movie *Fatal Attraction*. [31] I would never follow you, call your home, or force you onto an examining table. My abstract thinking, my little fantasy, is really just an innocent schoolgirl crush. Once again, I am drawn to the authoritative figure. I want to be your dearest child.

Now what? I suppose you want to consult with Deepak Chopra. Your golfing buddy is right. If you are bonding with Deepak, someone needs to medicate you.

I am thankful to enjoy these sensations and the fact that I

am alive to receive the benefits. It is something you and I can joke about. Along with mad, my secret infatuation has probably added several more months to my longevity.

A sexual relationship is not what I desire with my man-doctor. But, oops, the Bible says I have already committed adultery by lusting. And reading about "the holiness of God gives me a clearer estimate of my own failings."[32] Yet I don't think of myself as a promiscuous, wanton woman, especially not in this scarred-up, lopsided, overweight body. I know I cannot turn a head anymore, which is a painful realization.

My passion is hard to describe on paper. Humans may not understand. But God knows my heart. Today's candid discussion with the Mighty Counselor brought me peace. And he loves it when I call on him in this way. He helped me understand my need for men in my life, specifically and currently, Alan S. Collin, M.D.

I am trying to fill a void. Daddy and my uncles are dead. I have no brothers. I cannot relate to my brothers-in-law, although I respect them. My husband and I interact as man and wife, as well as best friends. However, I crave varied male influence in my life, and I am of the belief that one person cannot fulfill all the needs of another.

Friendships with men are easy. You don't have to worry about cycles, mood swings, or competitiveness—all of which are typical of female companionship. (And right here Neal offers his observation: women are basically deceitful people.) But society and the old-time religion frown upon the practice of platonic relationships among men and women, especially married people. They say platonic relationships flirt with trouble. Why is this? My daughter defies society's theory. She knows how to enter into relationships with commitment but states clearly her men friends are vital and there is no room for jealousy. Caryn exercises freedom to be herself. When I grow up, I want to be like my daughter.

So I don't need sex, and a platonic friendship with the doctor is taboo. What I specifically and currently need from

Alan S. Collin, M.D.—are you ready for this?—is big brotherhood. Do you remember when I said to you once, "I need something from you, but I don't know what it is." To which you playfully inquired, "Is it bigger than a bread box?"

You crack me up. Yes! That's it, a big brother in a white coat who is bigger than a breadbox.

Now that I have defined my need, what can be done about it? Nothing changes. There is no time for sibling behavior in a cubicle should you even accept the assignment.

What would I do with my new big brother if I could steal him away from the office for a few hours? I would be an embarrassment to you on the golf course. You'd be bored stiff with my hobbies. Could we harmonize on clarinet and bassoon? Ooh, that is a scary thought. I can't picture you dancing in the surf or power walking beside me. I suppose I could meet you for breakfast at Marie's Gourmet Kitchen or take in a movie, though we'd probably make the front page of the hometown news. Would we help each other move, or attend children's bar mitzvahs, graduations, weddings? No, probably not.

But I would be so honored if you needed me and called on me on occasion. Bill Withers places that thought in my head when he sings "Lean on Me." Alan S. Collin, M.D., lean on me, when you're not strong, and I'll be your friend, I'll help you carry on. You just call on me, brother, when you need a hand.[33] We all need somebody to lean on—even strong, confident doctors.

There's not much chance of interaction outside the office, so let us head back to the cubicle. I am sweet sixteen and you are, well, big-brother age. I easily crawl up on your lap and tell you every fear, every dream, every secret. And you divvy out the protection, the compassion, wisdom, and teasing of a big brother. I am reassured you will sit there with me for as long as it takes. The office visit ends when I hop down and say, "Thanks, I feel better. You can see your next patient now."

Daydreaming comes to a dead stop. I am still just another cancer patient and there are identical creatures banging on the exam room door. It is three deep out there, each one carrying a satchel full of whimsy, fantasy, and drug-induced, abstract thoughts.

I fear delicate feelings have no place in the oncology office, despite what you all advertise. Forget about being special in the doctor's eyes. The body is just a machine. The cancerous body is simply a broken-down machine. Get out the needle-nose pliers, the wrench, the hammer. Tighten up that valve from where tears flow or we'll see corrosion. Tears are a dime a dozen in the oncology office.

Is this how it goes? God, I hope not. I wish I could say I don't need any silly old doctor to make me feel better. But I do. I especially need the silly part.

While typing all this down, reckoning and reasoning myself onto page after page, God beckons me to drive out to meet him at the beach. It is raining. No dancing. I will wear my rain poncho, take my lawn chair, and plant myself in a dripping sea breeze where tears blend in and wash away. A beach sign reads "No Lifeguard on Duty," but God is my lifeguard and he is always on duty. His power revives.

Man, doctor, brother—whoever you are: if you write a new medical textbook about me, be sure to list stomping around, frank talk with God, angry letter-writing, and dripping sea breeze as good tonics for bronchitis. I am on the road to recovery.

> Dear brothers, is your life full of difficulties and temptations? Then be happy, for when the way is rough, your patience has a chance to grow. So let it grow, and don't try to squirm out of your problems. For when your patience is finally in full bloom, then you will be ready for anything, strong in character, full and complete.
>
> James 1:2-4 (TLB)

Looking back, I have yearned for big brotherhood from other

influential men in my life. It never works out. What is the matter with you people? My big brother search continues. Or does it? No, I shall look no further. My spirit is kin to yours for some reason. I choose you. I think Mom and Daddy would choose you even though you misbehave and screw up once in a while. Big brothers do.

Can you rededicate yourself as my big brother this Chanukah?

Do I sign my name to this one?

Connie

Connie—#25561—full of difficulties and temptations, but trying not to squirm out of my problems.

Friday, January 29, 1999

Dear Administrator of Life:

If ever I needed a warm embrace from you, it is today. But my appointment is not for several weeks.

Did I tell you I am a Methodist? We Methodists sing, "I believe for everyone who goes astray, someone will come, to show the way..."[34] I blew the chance to be that someone who shows the way. Thirty minutes might have made a difference.

For one whole year I have faithfully walked or semi-faithfully danced on South Hudson Island. And I've shared with you the abundant treasures I find there, such as well-being, vitality, and the very breath of God. Beauty and song reign, no matter what...until yesterday, Thursday, January 28, 1999. A gentleman shot and killed himself at my private oasis while I walked with joy just a few yards away.

No bird sang.

My walking/dancing regimen was interrupted briefly by an upper respiratory infection. But I returned to Seaside Park yesterday afternoon. Afternoon is not my assigned time slot, yet it worked with the day's agenda. What a welcome delight to get back into a cadence on the boardwalk. I don't think I've ever seen such rich, vibrant colors—in the sky, in the ocean, in the greenery. Everything about our seaside reached out to greet me. Perhaps a half-dozen older people milled around the park. They all appeared to be pleasant, happy people. What a glorious day! Thanks be to God for designing this magnificent natural wonder and leading me to it in his *perfect* time.

I rounded Seaside Park's south end, finishing the first lap. An older woman trailed close behind. Her frame, hairdo, and smile reminded me so much of my mother that a sentimental tear moistened my cheek. We were steps apart in the shelter house when a startling shot rang out. I thought it sounded like a BB gun. A flock of birds fluttered nervously in the direction of the sound. Thick, tall sea grasses blocked our view of the beachfront at that moment. My mommy-look-alike and I both missed a step and wondered aloud who would shoot BBs at our seagull friends. But we didn't investigate. We shrugged and parted ways. She headed home and I hoofed on down the boardwalk, trying to keep on schedule. I needed to pick up my son at 3:00 p.m. sharp.

My power walk finished and I strolled to the end of the beach access for deep breathing. There my eyes witnessed a slow-motion melodrama I cannot seem to shake. Deep breathing ceased. All breathing ceased.

A beach walker struggled to drag a body up out of the surf. For a split second, through my tears, I convinced myself a large, black, shiny fish floated ashore. But this large black shiny fish had two human legs. I wanted to run closer and run away at the same time, yet my running shoes were cemented to the wooden boardwalk. For the longest time it was just the three of us: the upright beachcomber hovering over a large, shiny, black [dead] fish in sea foam of unusual color, and frightful me, frozen stiff to the boardwalk. My eyes scanned the coast for human help only to find deserted beach for miles either way. All those happy, pleasant folks disappeared out of sight. And no bird sang.

I summoned up enough nerve to shout to the beachcomber, "What happened?"

He responded, visibly shaken, "I don't know, but the guy has a bloody hole in his head. I think he is still breathing."

The gunshot. Oh, my God. I remembered the gunshot from moments before. Now I knew it was no blasted BB gun, but an authentic revolver. Did someone shoot him, and if so, where is he or she at this moment? Or did this distraught, desperate creature thoughtfully put on his wet suit and pull the trigger himself?

It was my nervous fingers that dialed 911 on the payphone

out by the street, and within minutes sirens, badges, equipment, questions, and well-meaning onlookers saying all the wrong things surrounded us. A weapon was retrieved from the surf.

I had to be clear of one issue fast. If I had responded immediately after hearing the shot, could I have saved his life? The officer in charge answered with an emphatic "No. He died instantly." I have to believe him. My next burning question is, if I had come by thirty minutes sooner, could I have talked him out of it, shown a better way? God only knows.

My rose-colored sunglasses fell off in this scuffle.

Why was he so sad?

Usually I heal myself of despair by writing, but today's severely jumbled thoughts do not come easy. Bear with me. The best I can do is spew fragments of disbelief and horror that pound inside my soul.

Folks die daily. Some choose their timing. My husband's point-blank comment is: "Many people, over the course of history, have committed suicide at the sea. This is not unusual. You didn't know him—get over it."

But not my sea. Not where beauty and peace rush in to heal me. Not in a place where I work with great effort to stay alive and nurture some vibrancy. Not while I am within earshot. God, forgive me. Earshot is a poor choice of words.

Once again, I hardly ever walk the beach in the afternoon. And the afternoon is five hours long. Why was I there at that exact moment? What's all this nonsense about God's perfect timing?

If I had stayed home yesterday—I don't read the newspaper—I would still be walking merrily along, never knowing a man shot himself on my beach.

I could have been at the other end of the boardwalk when he pulled the trigger, and with the wind blowing from the north, his gunshot and last breath would have gone unnoticed by me. Some days I don't take time to deep breathe after walking. Yesterday could have been one of those days.

I've laid claim to that particular twelve-foot section of Seaside Park. Why did he choose to take his life on my personal property? I begin and end my walking regimen at this very point. He was floating dead in the exact place where I float, I pray, and get filled up with hopeful energy.

My heart aches for this stranger.

"Why was he so sad? And why did God factor me into his puzzle?"

I forced myself to go there and do my regular thing this morning. I didn't think it wise to go alone, but not one friend was available, so I did go alone, and I cried each step of the way. No sign of death or despair lingered with the elements, though. The only remnant of strife was between me and the seagulls. We looked at each other with an inexpressible, painful secret.

My ultimate pain comes from wondering what happens to this poor man's soul. I've heard more than once that if you take your own life, you can never get away from what's bothering you and God is not available for comfort.

"No, no. Please, God, hold this man's soul in the palm of your sturdy, loving hand. Show him all the beauty, and love, and acceptance he apparently could not find here on earth, and please bring peace and comfort to his family."

Dr. Collin, I know you hate death talk. I am sorry. What makes me want to spill my guts out to you, anyway? You are a medicine man who is not interested in or capable of answering repetitive deep questions.

But why, oh why was this gentleman so sad?

No bird sang. Neither did I dance.

Connie

Tuesday, March 2, 1999

Happy Birthday to My Handsome, Humorous Medicine Man (a few days early),

My gift to you: a thoughtful interlude.

Why do I often think of you? Office visits are far between now, yet the command in your voice coaches me to dream and dance, to breathe ocean mist and plant seeds on a daily basis. Your funny stories run through my head like a continuous cartoon strip. I laugh at inopportune moments. White cells multiply right there on the spot.

I see bright, sparkling stars in your eyes one December morn. You talk about your three sons. Santa is on my mind and, for a moment, you are him. (His eyes, how they twinkle). I am just about to crawl up onto your lap for a long winter's nap. Isn't that the way the story goes? Now I wonder…are the stars in your eyes or in mine? There I go again…thinking.

Why do I often think of you? A picture of you standing in the hallway drinking a Coke like an ordinary man bothers me. Didn't I just touch the hem of your cloak and receive your healing power? Shouldn't you be perched on holy ground, behaving as royal lineage?

Why do I often think of you? Who are you, anyway? I know nothing about you. I only know the man I created you to be.

You are my Tevye (Topol)[35] and my *Patch Adams*[36] with the red rubber nose. You are the brave daddy in *Deep Impact*.[37] You slay the beasts of the business and ride away in crisp, white coating. Dare I compare you to the Messiah and my husband, whom I occasionally equate to be one and the same? Yes, you resemble my very own husband in stature and wit. Groovy, huh?

You have all the indications of a brass man, yet claim to be a woodwind. You are a golf enthusiast for whom I have no intelligent questions, and always, forever, you are the tireless stand-up comedian.

But who are you, really...besides all this? And why must I think of you so often?

Another Jewish hero occupies my thoughtful inner chambers. Jesus of Nazareth is his name. He too is in the business of healing spirits, saving lives, telling stories. The God of Israel sent him to save me, the Gentile...me, the sinner. When I worship the God of Israel and thank him for doing so, I think of you.

This Jesus lives inside me now, today, in the very place where I think of you. Come. Meet with him on the park bench of my soul. Discuss your mutual livelihood. Exchange stories of healing miracles. Laugh with him. And when your conversation ends, shake his hand as friends do. You will notice the nail scar and thank him for another matter.

Why do I often think of you? Is it worldly intrigue or am I on a Divine mission? One Jew, one Gentile, one King embraced within my heartbeat.

I accept. The seeds you wish me to plant...are for you.

God of Israel, please hold this ordinary man in your extraordinary hands.

With love,

Connie

Connie

Tuesday, April 20, 1999

Hello:

Arimidex seems to work well for me. My six-month scans look clean as a whistle. Yippee!

That's not the most important part of today's business, though. I want to point out a subject missing from the *Chemotherapy and You*[38] booklet. Please take notes. Folks should know their behavior is normal.

One of the residual side effects of chemotherapy padded with steroids is raiding the refrigerator at 3:16 a.m. The cows in the pasture behind our house complain of glaring kitchen lights every night. Moo!

My neighbor cancer buddy and I are bonded together with middle-of-the-night snacking. I am up front about my habit; she's in denial. We talked about this at the ball field the other day. I chuckle at the thought that she and I are in our kitchens at the same hour. I wonder what she is eating and how much. But I feel sad for her. If she is in true denial, she cannot enjoy herself.

I crave sweets. Rarely do I get up and search for protein or salt. I am hooked on Publix Heath Bar Frozen Yogurt and often take the carton and a spoon to my bed in the dark. That way I can eat until satisfied with no regard for calories, fat content, or any other convicting details in the black square on the back of the carton. My other favorites are peanuts or peanut butter, raisins, almonds, cake, cookies, coconut out of the bag, fruit juice, Jell-o, pudding, orange slice candies, and marshmallows. Did I mention candy bars?

With an open container of Heath Bar Frozen Yogurt and a spoon, I can be fairly quiet so Neal's snoring doesn't miss a beat. If there is any tearing of packages, I move into the guest bedroom at the other end of the house so as not to disturb the family...or get caught.

Pretty bad practice, I admit. How can I boast to you or counsel others about cleaning up the diet? Okay. Next time I come in whining about steroid weight gain and it being all your fault, I give you permission to twirl around, get right in my face (something you do well), and remind me of my middle-of-the-night snacking.

I broke this weakness for a while, a short while, and drank only water. But it's bad again, and each time I get up to go to the bathroom, three or maybe four times a night, my widening frame saunters toward the refrigerator and cupboards, salivating. This creates a new meaning for refrigerator magnet. There are worse habits, I suppose. You and Neal can be thankful I am not driving over the bridge to Archibald's Bar in the wee hours.

Envision my neighbor and me in the dark nights. Me, fully awake and aware, munching away; her, feasting with one eye open, and then collecting wrappers *the grandchildren* left on her nightstand! Oh, yeah. The pasture and the cows butt up to her property too.

Research shows cancer/chemo patients peer into their refrigerators in the middle of the night around the world. Refrigerator lights ease the dark emptiness of our tummies, but also our hearts. Health concerns don't seem quite as scary during this habit. God must be amused. And cows moo all over the globe.

Regards from the country,

Connie

Connie

• • •

Tale by the Sea

The more wrappers on my nightstand, the more often I need to drive over to the beach for a workout.

Since Neal and I built our home in the country with the cows and we are country people, coastal scenery fascinates me. I fantasize about lifestyles on the island.

South Hudson islanders do not work for a living. They stay up late carousing; sleep late nursing hangovers; revive themselves in the rhythmic tide; surf like they are still twenty-one; ride bikes honking horns or ringing bells for clearance; and when the sun goes down, they entertain. Well, they call it entertaining. Country people call it carousing, especially if Jim Beam, Johnny Walker, and Jack Daniels are invited.

In one of my fantasies, I secure a tiny abode—an efficiency apartment within a stone's throw of the sounds, scents, and laziness of endless summer. I, too, can be an unemployed South Hudson islander, except I cannot stay up late carousing because I turn into a pumpkin at 9:30 p.m., and I can't sleep late because I get a headache—a regular headache, not a hangover headache. I have and can very well revive myself with the power of a rhythmic tide; however, I'd have to exchange the surfboard for one of those red-canvas wave riders and there would be no mistake that I am fifty-something, riding that wave. No way should I try to pedal a bicycle and ring a bell at the same time. I never liked to entertain. And with the cocktails you serve in the chemo room, it would be lethal to meet up with Jim or Johnny or Jack, right?

Well...I should probably stick to country life with the cows.

Monday, August 16, 1999

Dear Fellow Pisces:

Our hot water tank works under strain. I've taken three hot showers in the last four hours. My theory is any disease or sadness can be washed off and I will be done with it. You, a Pisces, should understand.

A bit of pain in the left chest wall convinced me to make an appointment with Dr. Cappelletti last Wednesday. He seems concerned about the small lump on my scar line and ordered an ultrasound. Apparently the two of you conversed and agreed this lump is probably malignant. I fear you are right. Now all of a sudden a bit of pain turns into a bundle of pain, and I get the sensation my chest cavity is filling up with bad cells. Cappelletti's nurse called this morning. She said ultrasound results were inconclusive. The surgeon wants to schedule another biopsy to be sure.

I swear. April's scans were clear and clean. How could I develop a problem so quickly?

Cut again, wait for results, and rack my brain with decisions. The nurse's phone call might as well be the first shovel of dirt. Why am I being a jerk now? Didn't I know this beast would get me? A while back I prepared myself for death and accepted the idea graciously. Look at me now. Pathetic.

Arimidex gave me an eighteen-month reprieve. I should give God thanks. Notice I do not call it *remission*. Remission reminds me of a grizzly bear in hibernation, gaining weight, ready to break loose stronger than ever. No. Remission and/or grizzly bears are not mentioned in this household.

"Calm down, Connie," you say. "Let us hear the pathology results before we jump out of the boat." Doc, would you jump out of the boat with me, really?

I sink in a swirl of endless questions. What is death like? How is it going to happen, exactly? Will I lay motionless like a vegetable for months or years? Or, if death is not immediately on my doorstep, what will you prescribe and how sick will it make me? What does my blood work look like? What alternative agents shall I start taking? When multiple treatments are used, how are we supposed to know what is effective and what is not? Whew. Isn't there something else I can do with my time? I am too young for this business.

Have I been a bad girl? Sorry, God. Sorry, Dr. Collin. You mutter to me, "Oh ye of little faith, why do you doubt?"

Clancy Barrish called last evening to share how Nanette died. That's one reason I've got death on the brain. Her passing turned out the best it could be. She slipped into a coma Saturday evening. Hospital staff took away the noisy machinery, gave her a bath, and arranged lovely flowers all around her. She rested there peacefully for twenty-four hours and took her last breath with best friends by her side. Way to go, Nanette.

I won't be that fortunate.

Today I wish I could lie down and get it over with. I told you my spirit was strong enough to endure anguish and misery. Well, guess what. I lied. I no longer want to see the pain in my husband's eyes. I don't want to hear what an inconvenience I am to my children. Friends and family members think I can beat anything, but they are sadly misinformed.

My biopsy is docketed for Friday, August 20.

No one listens to my wailing other than you.

My vessel is buffeted by the waves. The wind is against it. My focus is off course. I am afraid. Am I kin to Peter?

Connie

. . .

Tale by the Sea

In the *NIV Encouragement Bible*, Dave Dravecky comments on Matthew 14:30-31. "Focusing continually on our circumstances accomplishes nothing. It doesn't change them; it only gives them the power to sink us. I think of the famous story of Peter's brief walk on the water. As long as he kept his eyes on Jesus, the water beneath him was as good as concrete. But '…when he saw the wind, he was afraid…' (v. 30) and began to sink. 'You of little faith…why did you doubt?' (v.31) Jesus asked after saving his soaked disciple from drowning. Peter didn't answer."[39]

Neither shall I answer your questions, Dr. Collin. The nerve of you, asking where my faith is, why I doubt! Just leave my sinking spirit alone. That's sinking not *stinking*, or maybe it is stinking. Whatever. The sky is heavy and overcast. The beach is deserted. No one walks on water today. I see no bathers or bikers. Archibald's outdoor restaurant and bar is dead at high noon. Sun worshippers apparently don't go out unless the sun is out to be worshipped. Plus they sure don't want to hear any one-breasted complaints by the seaside. Did I dance today? No dancing. I am too wrinkled from three hot showers.

Tuesday, August 24, 1999

Good Evening, Dr. Collin:

Last Friday, Dr. Cappelletti ran after me with his knife again. Or was it a jigsaw? Good words, great words of hope spilled from him. He said to me, while sawing, that he really couldn't find what he went after. "Where is it?" He excised a good amount of tissue anyway. Ouch, one more time.

The good surgeon himself called this afternoon at 2:20 p.m. Pathology on the tissue in question proves clean! No malignancy! I could hear cheering chants in the background, and God knows it is music to our ears. It's the first bit of favorable news Cappelletti has been able to give us. This is a personal victory for all involved. Small and large miracles *do* happen. God is still in the miracle business. I should never second-guess him.

The best place to mend itchy stitches this evening is under our ol' oak tree.

Neal winks at me while he trims the bushes. Our dog, Bob, has a smile on his snout, a spring in his step. He protects me from lizards and squirrels. With paper and pencil in hand, I jot down goals.

Goal No. 1: I will strive to be the kind of person my dog already thinks I am.

Goal No. 2: I will see you next Tuesday. You may take a peek at my clean, clear, healthy chest. No charge.

Goal No. 3: I think I'll climb the Highland Trail at Glacier National Park with a woman named Arlene.

Connie

• • •

Tale by the Sea

I drove out to the beach this morning for a healing breath of sea mist. Seaside Park looked especially green and lush. I know why. Good news was on its way.

The supervisor for the ground maintenance crew at Seaside Park is a Jamaican man with a hook for an arm. His other weapon is a power chainsaw. This one-armed bandit/pirate scared the heebie-jeebies out of me back when I first started visiting the beach alone. I remember fumbling for my keys and racing to my car. He was there the next day, and the next day my heart pounded just as loud. Gradually I noticed his uniform and what he drives—a county maintenance vehicle. I later learned he is the daddy of one of my daughter's classmates and a true man of God. Now I greet and meet this hook and chainsaw operator on a first name basis. Picture a one-breasted gal conversing with a one-armed man in the midst of God's lush creation.

Knives and jigsaws, hooks and chainsaws no longer scare me.

Tuesday, October 26, 1999

Dear Doctors, Nurses, Staff:

Thank you for taking gentle care of my friend Nanette Barrish.

You provide a safe harbor for each patient. At appointment time we pull up to the dock flat and lost, you tinker away, then we're turned back out to sea, whole and focused. We arrive in a weakened state but leave at full throttle.

It's a place where we can safely learn from each other. Words aren't always necessary. I remember watching Nanette breeze through a Taxotere treatment, supposedly fearless, definitely tan and spunky, while I whimpered with side effects in the next room. She put me to shame. That picture of her was worth a thousand reasons to exit my pity party and lace up my dancing shoes. And so it was, and I did, and I will.

"Teach us to number our days and recognize how few they are; help us to spend them as we should" (Psalm 90:12, TLB).

Nanette loved adventure, from the mountaintops to the bottom of the ocean. I cherish two photos of Nan, one of her diving down into the depths of the ocean and one of her on the tip-top of a snowy mountain. Nanette definitely spent her few days as she should.

I present to your office an afghan of sea creatures. It reminds me of Nanette. Use it to keep your chemo patients warm. When the time is right you can share stories of our courageous deep-sea diver/mountain climber. Her spirit continues to inspire. All it takes is an example or an idea. You'll have chemo patients bounding out of those chairs, getting busy with life at full throttle.

I like coming to my safe harbor for reinforcement. Nanette did too. Because of your high degree of dedication, our bodies and souls rise above this illness no matter what our finish line looks like.

With grateful heart,

Connie

Connie Titus

Tuesday, November 9, 1999

Dear Dr. Collin:

On August 31 you released me for twelve weeks, providing October's CT scans are in my favor. I argued, "Thank you, no." Clear scans or not, a cancer survivor with decreased certainty in her life requires guidance, fortification, and a howdy-do from her oncologist on a frequent basis.

However, I agreed to go twelve weeks on my own. The truth is I am never really on my own. Doctors may abandon ship, but God keeps on steering. The Lord spoke to Joshua and the Lord speaks today, to Connie Titus on Windemere Drive. "As I was with Moses, so I will be with you; I will never leave you nor forsake you" (Joshua 1:5, NIV).

So I tried your twelve-week plan—six weeks for port flush, three months to see your smiling face. CT scans took place on Thursday, October 21. Gosh, look what happened. One more time, "I am no good on my own."

The scan of my head reveals a small, new one-centimeter dark spot in the brain. Neal says he could have saved us money. According to him, there are numerous dark spots in my brain. It doesn't appear to be a mass, or a clot; nor is there any evidence of a stroke, which is a relief. A further exam, MRI, showed no highlight as it would a malignancy. Scientific jargon reads, "Right frontal lesion likely from focal Encephalomalacia of undetermined etiology."

That's a fancy way to say I own a brain malady of unknown nature in my right forehead. The word unknown is strangely comforting. You conferred with the radiologist at length. The two of you are still baffled.

Let me remind you, I am not your run-of-the-mill textbook gal.

I love the way you instigate a belly laugh over something serious. According to you, in order to thoroughly diagnose the malady, you must first take my face off, look at this thing, and ask me what to do about it. Cute. Do you mind if I pass on face removal?

Neal's dear, funny friend suggests it is a microchip to define wild animals. I'll bet you are sorry you didn't think of that.

So I am walking around with a microchip in my brain. It doesn't prevent me from stirring a soup pot, folding boxer shorts, or taking control of the remote. God must have something important for me to do here on earth. Let us pray I can discern exactly what it is.

It's my sneaky way to see you more often than every twelve weeks. You don't want me wandering around, unsupervised, with a microchip in my brain, do you?

Love,

Connie

Connie, with an undermined etiology

• • •

Tale by the Sea

I am using my new microchip to define wildlife at the beach. Last week moon jellies washed up on shore. Have you ever seen one? What a peculiar species. Clear, jellied, round, and flat creatures, some of them as large as twelve inches in diameter. They have a bright pink ring around the edge. In the center is a pocket of four egg-like sacs. Gross. The lifeguard warns they are poisonous. I wonder for what purpose they are created. And these moon jellies look at me and wonder for what purpose I am created.

I also witnessed my first fresh set of sea turtle tracks. Large sea turtles lay their eggs on the beach at night. Turtle Mothers walk along the shore before dawn, locate fresh tracks, rope off the nesting area, and mark the date on a stake. That way they can judge the gestation period and possibly be available to assist the tiny ones back into the sea. I smiled about the *set* of tracks and mused over turtle romance—Daddy Turtle accompanying Mom to bury her eggs. How gullible I am. Neal explained those are Mom's tracks on the way up, and Mom's tracks on the way back.

The sign on the lifeguard tower says "Lifeguard Only— Keep Off," but I have cancer. I can do what I want. I climb up past the sign and have a seat. From there my microchip does its job.

Friday, December 10, 1999

Dr. Collin: Holiday Greetings (NOT):

Whatever you do, don't ask about dancing or daybreak because I lie still, flimsy, brittle. I find no comfort in a soft bed. Jesus sits in the chair beside me, his head in his hands. He died on the cross for me and I act like it wasn't enough. I beg him to stop wasting time with me and put his efforts into my family, make *them* light in spirit, supply *their* needs.

Why the crummy attitude? I succumb to a normal, natural, seasonal flu. That's all. Cancer days haunt me even though there's no evidence at this time. The dark spot in my brain turned out to be nothing, so I can't blame that.

Titus Family Oppression rings loud and clear. *Here we go again; Mom is in bed. What good is she?*

Our daughter is hurting, confused, lost, and alone in Gainesville. She needs me, but I can't go to her. I am not even able to say the right things over the phone. Our son harbors anger. We cannot afford the toys he thinks he needs. "What do you mean we can't buy fireworks for the Millennium? Why don't you just go to work, Mom—all my friends have two working parents."

My husband toils tirelessly in Santa's woodshop—my idea, not his. He untangles endless strands of Christmas lights, followed by digging through towering piles of clean laundry for one stinkin' (but clean) pair of underwear. Yet he utters not a mumbling word. Gifts need wrapping, boxes need mailing, but first, someone should probably shop. Bah, humbug.

Inside decorations wait to be placed; swirls of dust encircle them. I cannot concentrate or see clearly. But I clearly see the bleach water stains on our windows. The garage is an obstacle course—bring in a backhoe. The cat desperately needs a flea bath. Our son's tuba quartet wants to come for practice and dinner. I hope the tuba quartet is not allergic to dust...or flea bags. Dinner? Who is cooking dinner?

My mother was sick all the time. I complained about the fact. Payback is a condition of torment.

Does what I do when I'm active balance out listlessness? Will my husband and children remember active goodness, if there is any, or will they remember lazy, sick, pathetic Mom? Where is my happy trust in the Lord, God? I shrink from trusting Him. I'll tell you one thing: depression trounces a family's Christmas spirit.

Oh, no, look at this. Authors of the Holy Bible have my number.

> Do not let this happy trust in the Lord die away, no matter what happens. Remember your reward! You need to keep on patiently doing God's will if you want him to do for you all that he has promised. His coming will not be delayed much longer. And those whose faith has made them good in God's sight must live by faith, trusting him in everything. Otherwise, if they shrink back, God will have no pleasure in them.
>
> Hebrews 10:35-38 (TLB)

God will have no pleasure in me if I don't straighten up and fly right. Dr. Collin, can you help me straighten up and fly right? My next office appointment isn't until Tuesday, December 21. You told me to call you if I need you. Which task do you prefer: backhoe operation in the garage, cat's flea bath, or cooking dinner for a tuba quartet? God have mercy. Oncologists don't know how to do any of this. The mental image of you trying is good for a cackle, though. Thank you.

Connie

Connie, guilty as charged

• • •

Tale by the Sea

No dance, no sunrise, no tale, no sea. I am shipwrecked until further notice.

Friday, January 28, 2000

Good Morning, A.S.C., M.D., Ocean Lover:

I am between office visits. Toss one more letter into the citrus box.

I approach the two-year mark on Arimidex, a drug thought *not* to help ER/PR negative bodies, yet scans prove clean. Side effects multiply over time. To date, I claim only sixteen of the twenty-six possibilities. Uh oh. Did that sound sarcastic?

I am thinking of you, knowing how much you love the water. I prescribe for you a happy new year.

The ocean: oh, my goodness. Beachcombing is an enticing career for this Pisces. I do, indeed, live on what I find. God created the seashore for me and he created me for the seashore. Too bad it took me nineteen years to come to such a conclusion.

There is a storm in the southeast, just off the shoreline. There is another storm in the northwest. Yet the two shall not meet in the middle where I dance.

The sun is shining on me, for me, around and through me. It shimmers and glitters on the water's surface. There is not another soul in sight. My Creator and I dance alone.

Even before Moses' time, God knew of Connie Beth Thompson Titus. He knew what my laughter would sound like. He declared game shows and heavy perfume would drive me bonkers. He knew whom I would love. He recorded dates when medical doctors would deliberate over poor test results. He designed my lively spirit to thrive regardless and splash onto others by means of (computerized) pen and paper. He knew I would visit with him at Seaside Park this morning, January 28, 2000, at 8:43 a.m. sharp, with thankful heart. And he deemed today the perfect day for Connie Titus to bloom where planted.

Blooming/blossoms, it is. Monocytes are on the rise. The water is refreshing on my feet. My roots dig down deep in wet sand. The air is clean and vibrant, causing rapid growth with many blossoms like a morning glory vine. I am growing so fast, I might turn inside out. (Ooh, Neal says he wants to see this.) In fact, let me check. Here today, in this gorgeous place, I claim only ten Arimidex side effects, not sixteen.

My Lord, what a morning! "O Lord, in the morning you hear my voice; in the morning I plead my case to you, and watch" (Psalm 5:3, NRSV).

Love from a buoyant Gentile friend,

Connie

Connie

```
      XXXXXXX
    XXXXXXXXXX
 XXXXXXXXXXXXXXXX
XXXXXXXXXXXXXXXXXXX
```

A breast cancer mastectomy
patient struggles uphill, both ways,
with self-image, sexuality, sensuality.
It is as if these things are cut off
and tossed aside with the breast
tissue. Even if a devoted,
loving, faithful husband
stands nearby with lust
in his eye and all the
encouragement he
can muster, she
falls short of sexy.
If only a stranger would
offer a wink or a second
glance. If only a friend of the
opposite sex would demonstrate
some intrigue…with a "want to" look
in his eye. A teasing attraction and some
good, honest flirting would certainly heal
these wounds. The "want to" part is what
we long for. No action. No reality. Just
a "want to." Yep. That would fix it!

```
XXXXXXXXXXXXXXXXXXXXXX
 XXXXXXXXXXXXXXXXXX
  XXXXXXXXXXXXXXXX
   XXXXXXXXXXXXX
    XXXXXXXXXXXX
    XXXXXXXXXXX
     XXXXXXXXXX
     XXXXXXXXX
      XXXXXXX
      XXXXXXXX
      XXXXXXXXX
      XXXXXXXX
      XXXXXXX
       XXXXXX
       XXXXX
       XXXXX
```

Connie

My sins are clearly seen here. Receive me with grace,
O Lord, just as I am. Amen.

Monday, March 6, 2000

Dr. Collin, My Friend,

Happy Birthday from a daydreaming patient. Jeanne may not want to tape this one to the family refrigerator. Not in plain sight, anyway.

Silent Eventide

She's been meeting him at the Dockside Inn every third Wednesday around 5:30 p.m. for the past three years. Her daydream never seems to progress beyond the calendar details. For the life of her, she cannot give form to what it is they do there...until now.

It's a dance, a long, lazy, simple two-step. The lights are low; the music is slow. They step back in time with Ella and Frank for a musical seduction. She is fully clothed, and he is as well, though his tie is loosened and his collar unbuttoned. The scent of him makes her dizzy for a moment. And for that moment, she has two breasts. Tensions of his workplace release into her nearness. Maybe he needs her too.

No words are spoken. No whispering, no expectations or questions. No funny stories. Not this time. No words are ever spoken. Not one word.

His cool, gray whiskers tickle her flushed cheek. Their fingers intertwine. Her tip-toeing stocking feet move in time, in sync, in rhythm with his deliberate, size ten steps. It is intimacy without a caress; a covenant without a kiss. She is happy just to dance with him.

The music ends. The music always ends. But their feet shuffle, lingering, until, at last, they stand still...very still.

Before parting, they walk to the pier, to witness the sun's disappearance. Is his tie still askew and his collar undone? Oh no. That is not for the world to see, it is a secret between he and she. Before stepping into the open, all is put neatly back together again.

And so they stroll to the water's edge, seeking their favorite bench. Not hand-in-hand or arm-in-arm like friends or lovers. But rather arm's length—hands in pockets—the body language of unavailable people.

They sit like strangers. Old Man River runs deep and wide as they muse over their regular, irregular, undefined togetherness. He winks. She blushes. Still the lips are silent.

As the red sun plunges into the town beyond the river, they simply share a day's end…on common ground, with zest, with understanding, and peace in the heart. Silent eventide is an unforgettable exchange.

Loving arms await them in different directions. Curious as it seems, her wholeness, his peace richly spill onto those they love best. And so it goes…until…another silent eventide.

Imagine asking a Jewish man to stand or sit next to another human being for slightly more than an hour without saying a word. Can he do it? Yes. In her daydreams, he can do it.

• • •

Years later, in reality, she visits the Dockside Inn searching for wedding guest accommodations. Ambience takes a dive. Flimsy hotel doors allow insects to come and go as they please. Her daydream no longer fits. No more dancing at Dockside Inn.

She now totes a huge, vibrant umbrella and two multi-positioned beach chairs to the surf's edge, hoping he will follow. It is a place where they can safely lose all track of time, from daybreak to eventide and back again.

Shall they converse at this new location? Will there be dancing? And how long will he be content before wandering down the shoreline to the next huge, vibrant beach umbrella?

I am close to you as you read this,

Connie

Connie

Tuesday, April 25, 2000

Alan S. Collin, M.D.,

It's nice to enjoy an uneventful office visit. CT scan films of head, neck, chest, abdomen, and pelvis look marvelous, check. Blood work in range, check. No new lumps or bumps, check. Same tolerable side effects with Arimidex, check. With any other physician this kind of encounter would be boring.

Not with you, though. Life stories and humorous illustrations, check.

I just love you. You set an example for me. Do other patients notice? I like the way you live your life. Family and fatherhood fill you up. The very thought of you makes me healthy, wealthy, and wise. I suppose there is much I don't know about you, but what I see and hear pleases me. I take big mental notes. Your zany humor is the first thing pulling me close, and you know how to lay attitudes on the line. Don't worry, be happy is your whistling motto. God's word lays it on the line, too. "So do not worry about tomorrow; it will have enough worries of its own. There is no need to add to the troubles each day brings" (Matthew 6:34, GNT).

Gee. Scripture indicates people have worries or troubles every day. I don't have any worries or troubles today. Do you?

Keep up the good work, Chief.

Your spirited strength, wisdom, and playfulness chase away pesky cancer cells and may end up getting me released from your care—the final outcome we've all been praying for, right? But I say *Yikes*! My port needs flushing every six weeks. On those days, do you mind if I tote in a lawn chair, park it in the hallway, and watch you in motion for a short while? I must take in a dose of you somehow, somewhere, in order to keep healthy.

I've got an idea. I will wear my pink lady volunteer smock, and you can put me to work filing, stapling papers, or making coffee. You and Nurse Nicole would be at arm's length, if and when I need you.

See you later, in some capacity,

Connie

Connie

• • •

Tale by the Sea

Seashells and rocks come in all shapes, sizes, and colors. I take remnants home. Today I smile for I found two body parts: a foot with a swollen, broken big toe and an uncircumcised penis. Remember, I am talking about rocks. Neal shows no excitement over today's treasures.

Tuesday, August 29, 2000

Dear Doctor Sir:

Neta and I dropped by today with a thank offering—an Okoboji Lake t-shirt and a resort guide advertising pristine golf courses in Iowa. Neta and her husband want to host one of your golfing retreats. Wish I could present you with a plane ticket too, but all you get today is a lousy t-shirt and an invitation.

Do not misconstrue this as a bribe. It's more of a buffer. Many of our church friends are under your care. They come by way of my referral. I have nightmares about you stepping into exam rooms where new patients demand a Connie Titus miracle, or else.

What can I say? Friends follow my intense survival story. They see my smiling strength and wonder if it is connected to your caretaking. In their time of oncology need, it's only natural they request a piece of your action. Apparently they put great stock in this passage: "In those days ten men from all languages and nations will take firm hold of one Jew by the hem of his robe and say, 'Let us go with you, because we have heard that God is with you'" (Zechariah 8:23, NIV).

All of these people truly understand that cancer is an individual venture and that the doctor is not in charge of miracles. At least I hope they do.

Please know I do not expect you to instantly heal them, produce nothing but good reports, or interrupt God's natural plan of life followed by death.

I do, however, enlist the warmth of your hand, request sweet/silly human stories to come sailing through that space in your teeth, and yes, I ask for your best-educated ideas where their individual ventures are concerned.

Just be yourself. I know you'll take good care of them.

Your character alone will benefit these people I love, whether it be for three years plus, or just several visits.

Thanks for watching over me and my friends.

May I pray for you? If you could ask for God's help this coming week, what is a specific need? No requests? Well, you missed your chance. I'll take it upon myself. "Dear Father of all mankind, please bless Dr. Alan S. Collin with balance, refreshment, joyful outbursts (his trademark), and if there are any demanding friends of Connie Titus' in the cubicles, please, please *protect him!* Amen."

Love,

Connie

Connie Titus

P.S. I do not charge for referrals.

Friday, November 17, 2000

Dear Primary-Care Physician of Mine:

Head, neck, chest, abdomen, and pelvis CT scans, and the regularly scheduled mammogram, PAP smear, and gynecological work-up show absolutely no malignancy. Am I one big miracle or what? But I have a bone to pick with you. Are you ready?

Even though your primary concern, my cancer, is confirmed quiet, aren't you still my primary doctor? When I am sick, I should notify you and let you handle it, correct?

For three weeks I have suffered with some kind of upper-respiratory junk. I refrained from bothering you and tried to fix it myself; after this length of time I am most sensitive to snowbird pressure. But hometown people crave your undivided attention, too. Our tug of war is why your crisp white coat gets tattered and torn.

Along about day nine I broke down and called your office. You ordered an antibiotic without any personal contact. After six days on the drug, there was no improvement. Do you know why?

Read an invisible footnote in the *Physician's Desk Reference*. "Medications prescribed for Connie Titus are ineffective without the doctor's hand on her shoulder, a famous funny story, or one of those 'resist me/push me away' neurological exercises."

Or maybe I needed one of those darned old steroid packs plus nebulizer treatments, which you finally prescribed for me, in person, on Tuesday.

In Tuesday's meeting, instead of a warm hand on my shoulder, empathetic eyes, or a funny story, you raked me over the coals for not speaking up about the severity of my condition and claimed you are not a mind reader. What? You cannot read minds? Sure you can. I've watched you sail through the office hallways tall and confident. Obviously you credit yourself with some kind of divine intervention, which would make reading minds a snap. When I contacted the office on day nine, why didn't you practice divination, read my mind, and pick up the phone? If you'd talked to me yourself, there would be no question as to the severity of my condition.

How I hate to complain about my favorite white-coated friend.

I am weak around the edges, but I did make it to the beach this morning. For this my family thanks you. Tomorrow, Saturday, if I am able, I will run by to rearrange your clinic door sign. I'll remove *Divine*, leave it plain old *Intervention*, and add the disclaimer *No Mind Reading*.

Connie

· · ·

Tale by the Sea

Twenty-one days absent from my beach, serious erosion takes place. Dredging equipment reigns. Sea grasses droop and play dead. Sad. Unrecognizable. Changed landscape just like me. Not a good place to dance.

Tuesday, March 6, 2001

Alan S. Collin, M.D:

Enclosed, for your birthday, is a photograph I took of day breaking over the ocean. The sun looks like a giant, bright star about to knock the dark cloud for a loop.

Speaking of stars, listen to this: Young children were interviewed about their thoughts on love. One little girl, Karen, age seven, said, "When you love somebody, your eyelashes go up and down and little stars come out of you." My goodness! What an eloquent expression from a young mind.

The eyelash part I know nothing about because I've not had any eyelashes to speak of, even pre-chemo. But the stars I identify with. My love for you is not a romantic love, but sometimes just as intense. Watch real close next time I am in the office. You will notice little stars coming out of me. Why not catch one, put it in your pocket, and never let it fade away? That way you'll be reminded of your good works with me and so many others.

A very happy birthday to you, my man-doctor!

Rambling on, maybe you should know I have written volumes about you, much of which is not yet on paper. You prove to be a fascinating subject…a star, in fact. Yes, you are a giant, bright star, knocking my dark cloud for a loop. "Shining star come into view…gives you strength to carry on. Make your body big and strong, future roads for you to pass…" [40]

With love,

Connie

Connie

Tuesday, May 1, 2001

Hi, Dr. Collin:

Medical reports on Connie Titus are clean, clear—positively super. Thanks for your influence. AstraZeneca should make me their new poster gal.

Our annual Relay for Life was fancy, festive entertainment. Banners, fireworks, line dancing—where were you?—luminaries, double-dip brownie sundaes—where were you?—and emotional energies in high gear made up one sensational evening. I, as a cancer survivor, appreciate the fundraising efforts of devoted teams. Brave people relayed all night for a cure.

One young survivor gave her story and outwardly announced loving her oncologist right there in front of God and everyone. She read a verse he had given to her, a poetic passage that improved her coping process. I don't think you are her doctor. The verse concept was you, but not the gift giving. However, if you are her oncologist, where is my gift? The beautiful fact is she felt comfortable declaring love into the microphone. Cancer survivors everywhere should profess love and appreciation to their oncologists on a regular basis. Pass me that microphone, please.

I try to keep a steady dose of adoration coming your way in these letters.

Survivors share a secret. Many times it's the oncologist who unveils the secret of life and living, as was the case with this young woman. You've done this with me time and time again. Handing me a poem is not necessary. I watch, I listen, I learn by your example. Thank you for imparting the secret to me in this manner.

For next year's event I suggest the following: Daytona's Relay Chapter invites area oncologists, surgeons, radiation oncologists, nurses, and staff members to walk the survivor's lap with them. Let's do it. Survivors put one foot in front of the other pressing forward with life. Trusty white-coated/blue-scrubbed doctors and nursing buddies back them up with their famous support—an impressive Kodak moment.

While I mused aloud whether or not you would participate in such an affair, Neal said you might, if enough patients apply pressure. Okay. If my idea flies with our local Relay administrators, consider me applying pressure today. I suppose you will arrange a tee time for that date. Of course no one knows the date yet. Besides, I would see through your makeshift excuse. Think about it. Get your staff revved up now.

I pray you are well and happy today, my friend. Find your relay shoes. "…let us run with patience the particular race that God has set before us" (Hebrews 12:1, TLB).

Stay tuned,

Connie

Connie

Thursday, July 12, 2001

Dear Dr. Collin:

God saved me, now I must save the world. That's the way it works. God lives and cares—I can be a witness, I can be a sign. "…you will be a sign to them, and they will know that I am the Lord" (Ezekiel 24:27, NIV). Scans are clear, blood work is in range, I look strong and healthy, so there is no reason why I can't get out there and show 'em how it's done.

I try. Townspeople certify me as cheerleader or spokesperson for anyone afflicted with disease, not just cancer. Friends seek my counsel and jokingly refer to me as Dr. Titus. Sick people observe my circumstance and response, and somehow their urge to leap from a tall building dissipates.

All joking aside, I jump into involvement with other cancer patients and search for their solutions. I love the fear out of them and guide them, like a good shepherd. The Bible instructs, "Be wise in the way you act toward outsiders; make the most of every opportunity. Let your conversation be always full of grace, seasoned with salt, so that you may know how to answer everyone" (Colossians 4:5-6, NIV). Grace I am mindful of. Whether or not I season my words with salt, you'll have to ask around.

Shepherding is serious business to me. My immediate family worries. Cultural barriers, co-dependent lifestyles, and those who repeatedly refuse my advice pose a challenge, and I either work with more diligence or lie awake agonizing. At times, this ministry is too big, too close. I fall limp and sick, reluctantly shutting myself off.

Today I gathered up all my grace and salt and set out to minister to a twenty-nine-year-old single mother who is losing ground. Sheryl is her name. Sheryl's arm is swollen up massively with a tumor; she is in an incredible amount of pain. Neither chemo nor radiation shrinks this tumor, yet she continues chemotherapy in quiet submission. She suffers in secret, asks no questions, has a strong faith but prays vaguely. My friend has not slept for three nights. She walks around and screams with a pillow in her mouth so she doesn't wake her mother or her young daughter.

I sat down beside Sheryl during chemo treatment (another oncology office). Connie Titus, whom folks regard as the woman with all the answers, turned incompetent. I stuttered while reading a list of hopeful ideas. It all sounded so foolish in the presence of Sheryl's pain. I offered to go to her home and read or sing to her, clean or cook, day or night. Chances are she will never ask.

How in God's name could I ramble on about coping skills while this sweet young woman squirmed in anguish? Silent handholding was what Sheryl needed…silent prayer, silent signs. Forget the grace and salt. I was not wise in the way I behaved today nor did I make the most of a shepherding opportunity. Please forgive me, Lord. Does my ministry stem from true love or survivor's guilt? Maybe someone else should carry the sign and save the world.

Connie

• • •

Tale by the Sea

Directly after Sheryl's appointment I drove over to the beach for big-time counseling. I met up with that man named Jesus. He initially came to town with me in mind, to save me from myself. I repeatedly need to be saved from myself. Today is a prime example.

My Divine Friend waited for me in the shelter house while I power walked. There is good reason for this. You see, he wears a long, white robe and sandals. A brisk walk on the wooden boardwalk would surely leave my Lord tangled up in a knot and blistered.

After my vigorous exercise, the Messiah and I sauntered down the shoreline, talking over this cancer thing, discussing my outreach to the world. He explained how I can best help myself and others. I, in turn, asked him a boatload of questions, putting my Christian upbringing to the test. Does he really go before us, preparing a way? Can we easily yoke ourselves with him, making our burdens light? Does he see potential in us, just as we are, even when we screw up the grace and salt situation? His resounding answer is *yes!*

The Lord walked and talked with me along life's narrow way on South Hudson Island, but why was there only one set of footprints?

He carried me.

Sunday, September 30, 2001

Good Morning, Man-Doctor:

I offer a simple hello from west of town along with a picture of morning's first light streaming through country pines in the pasture.

Did anything weird or wonderful happen to you Saturday, September 22? I often think of you, but usually my Alan S. Collin thoughts are spurred on by humor or song. On Saturday, September 22, I experienced shocking emotional flashes of your character, all day long, with no prompting. They have bothered me all week. I hope you are not in any trouble. Is everything all right?

Six-month scans are scheduled for Monday, October 8. We will see or hear from you shortly thereafter. Until then, stay safe.

With love and thanksgiving,

Connie, a curious country cowgirl

Thursday, January 24, 2002
Hand-Delivered

Good Morning, Dr. Collin,

Today is my birthday. Yes, I am still a Pisces. Today is my other birthday, and I'm in a mood to celebrate.

January 24, 1997, was the first day of the rest of my life. On that day, God created in me (gave birth to) a new spirit. That new spirit is five years old today. Five years is a milestone of relief for every cancer survivor. And according to those CT scan films of October, I have kicked cancer's butt.

January 24, 1997, felt like the first day of death, but I see clearly now. I see cleansing and healing from the inside out… a birthday and baptism all rolled into one. "…I had sprinkled clean water on you, for you will be clean…I will give you a new heart—I will give you new and right desires—and put a new spirit within you" (Ezekiel 36:25-26, TLB).

Folks look at me like I've got two heads when I say my cancer is a gift—a gift straight from the Father's hand. The passage above would make more sense to you if you knew me pre-cancer. But we won't go there today. We probably will not go there ever. I do not want to be responsible for all fourteen of your hairs standing on end. Just trust me. My cancer is a gift.

In my case, God sprinkles salty ocean water. And the clean, new heart/spirit and right desires are exactly what take place as I type this letter. God, in all his mystery, works for our good. Don't doubt this for a moment, sir.

Visions of sparklers on an ice cream cake dance through my head this morning, so I will stop by the grocery to buy one, drive towards the vast glorious sun shining in the east, and eat it all by myself.

On second thought, why don't you meet me there? Come on, Doc, play hooky. You are a contributing factor in this five-year birthday. I'll bring an extra spoon. We must eat ice cream cake very fast at the beach, so you'll be back to work in no time.

Oops, too late. While you were reading this letter, I had to go ahead and eat your half. Have a nice day anyway.

With love,

Connie

Connie Beth Thompson Titus

Wednesday, March 6, 2002

Happy Birthday, Alan S. Collin, M.D.:

Possessively, I claim you as handsome hero for one-breasted gals. Today I realize breast-cancer survivors are just one small part of your big picture. I now acknowledge you, my good man, as fearless leader of many tribes: the Hysterectomites and/or the Oophorectomites, better known as the Hystericals; the Colostomers, Lymphaticoes, and Prostatitanians; the Lobeless, Melanomanites, and Hemostatic-lass and lassies; and let's not forget the Brainlesionaires or Bilirubinites and probably a whole host of primitive clans I have not yet investigated.

Can you tell I am studying the Old Testament/Hebrew Scriptures and having some fun with it? Now if God is not offended, I will be safe in my fun.

All cancerous tribes come to you with bags, tubes, beepers, and whistles, or in my case, fake suppleness. Multiple frenzies, oddities, and incessant necessities complete the package.

You never miss a step, despite all this jazz. Taking our hands securely into yours, you carry our baggage and lead the way down the ominous trail into the jungle or into the desert. When darkness approaches, you help us set up camp, taking night watch until the fire goes out. You are faithful and true.

At one time or another, you so carefully deliver every patient to his or her personal oasis, the plateau at the edge of the trail. This place is distinctly different for each person. My oasis takes up residence at the seaside. Do you recall the exchange between us?

You sit beside me, on the right, in the taller authoritative chair. From there you impart a love for life as day breaks; you point to the stirring water and the constant incoming tide; you offer breadcrumbs to seagulls and urge me to soar high and higher with them; you voice the possibilities of joy beyond the horizon; and true to your character, our plateau encounter does not end without splashing and horseplay. Then we simply sit together silently. The sum total is (if you will) the very love of Jehovah himself. Through your splashing, your hand-holding and solidity, and in your orders to pack up my bedroll and fly high with the seagulls, I hear his still, small voice coaxing me to get on with it.

All tribes celebrate your birth today, Alan S. Collin, M.D. We thank God he put you together in such good fashion. Since the beginning of time, our names and needs were clearly written in his trusty Record Book; it was God's idea that you should come to our rescue.

Happy, happy day! Visualize your motley crew doing birthday cartwheels with our bags and whistles. Uh oh, my fake suppleness just fell out of its pocket. A beachcomber will find a thrilling, unique treasure in the sand today…a silicone breast.

Signed,

Connie

Connie—your clean, clear, cancerless IBC miracle woman sitting in the chair beside you

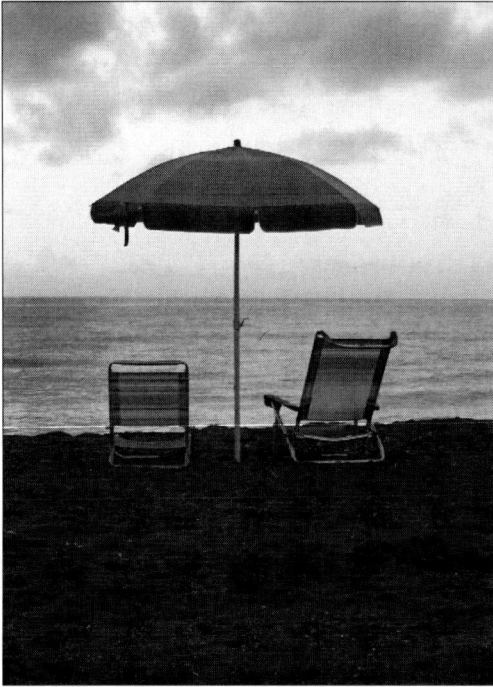

Patient Connie's campsite on her plateau. "...he orders his angels to protect you wherever you go. They will steady you with their hands to keep you from stumbling against the rocks on the trail" (Psalm 91:11, TLB). God sent a doctor-angel to steady Patient Connie so she will not strike her foot against any stone on the trail. "See the way God does things and fall into line" (Ecclesiastes 7:13, TLB). Patient is thankful her doctor-angel sees the way God does things and falls into his line of action.

Courtesy of Photographer Caryn Gonzalez

Saturday, May 25, 2002

Dear Dr. Collin:

The Titus Family wishes you Happy Thanksgiving in May. Enclosed is a musical gift.

Two weeks ago our only son ushered me down the center aisle of our church as Mommy of the Bride. Spectacular doings. Professionals predicted I would never see the day. I blew those predictions right out of the water as I sailed elegantly by family and friends who whispered "Wow!"

Our daughter, Caryn, and her groom, Jaime E. Gonzalez, Jr., burned this CD for wedding favors. It is their favorite love song collection. Caryn and Jaime show rich appreciation for the big-band sound and we are pleased. You will chuckle over a couple of their selections.

Track #1 is the trombone solo Jaime played to his bride during the ceremony. Our son-in-law is a professional musician who plays with jazz artists all over Florida. Ladies swooned and melted in their pews. A full trombone choir backed him up, including our son, Ron. "Double wow!"

Neal and I chose Jaime for Caryn. Yep, this was an arranged marriage. Actually we gave our daughter a choice of two trombone players: Jaime or their good buddy Kent. Kent disqualified himself by marrying Lucy, a French horn player, and it was at their wedding that Caryn and Jaime's six-year friendship rolled over into romance. *Yes!*

Now, Dr. Collin, my dear man, I order you to dance. Slip this CD into your home sound system and dance your wife around the island in your kitchen, if you have one. Kick up your heels, but be careful. Remember, you are over fifty. Do not fall, break a hip, and blame it on me.

Thanksgiving in May is a perfect season to dance and rejoice. You and God collaborate, elongating my life. You commanded me to dance, God invented the time and place, provided my strength and desire, and blessed us with a beautiful dancing celebration—our daughter's wedding. One more time: "Wow!"

Love from one dancing, rejoicing Mommy of the Bride,

Connie

Connie

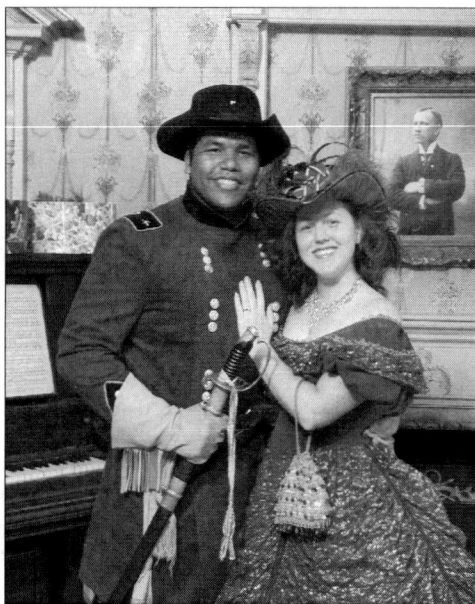

Engagement photograph and CD cover of Patient Connie's vintage daughter. Caryn, and her groom, Jaime Enrique Gonzalez, Jr. An arranged marriage.

Courtesy of Instant Ancestors Photography Studio

Friday, July 26, 2002

Dr. Alan S. Collin:

What a nifty early morning greeting. Neal opened up the newspaper to show me an acknowledgement and photo of you. Your partners, staff, and family congratulated you on twenty years of service on Florida's east coast. May patients chime in too? It is truly an honor to point to your picture and say, "I know him."

There is that boyish grin. I am partial to the space between your teeth from where laughter and wisdom ring through, mostly in the same breath. I have been a sucker for gray beards all my life. Nice, very nice. And, are those bright, sparkling stars in your eyes…the kind women write about?

You own *the look* that causes white cells to stand up tall and strong.

That same look almost got me into trouble at the supermarket a week ago. I found myself gazing…okay, staring at a distinguished gentleman with *the look*. He was just minding his own business, trying to choose a magazine from the empty checkout counter two rows over. I guess he felt my inquisitive eyes, for he looked up, right at me, right into my stare. Oh, my God! I blushed while fumbling with my checkbook. The clerk bothered me with the total of my order and I almost snapped, "Not now. Can't you see I'm busy?" But I did attempt to pay for my groceries with some degree of maturity. By that time, *the look* had abandoned his reading material search. Another long gaze followed him out of sight down aisle four.

Was *the look* a figment of my imagination, or did I make his day? It doesn't matter. What matters is tall, strong white cells parading out of the grocery store with a smile and a song.

The carryout boy wasn't too happy when I asked, "Where did I park? Which vehicle is mine? What's my name?"

I thank God for creating *the look* and I thank and praise him for creating eyes, souls, and white cells that respond to *the look*. Do you want to hear another tidbit? My husband has *the look*. The two of you share stature and witty composition and oh, those alluring gray whiskers. Between you two guys I am liable to hike mountain trails.

Alan S. Collin, M.D., Neal and I are both proud of you. May our tender, creative God bless you and motivate you for another twenty years of mission work.

Love,

Connie

Connie

P.S. You'll be relieved to know I did find my car in Publix parking lot, I remembered my name, and I drove home to the right house. Will you please jot the following in my chart: Tall, strong white cells parade, smile, and sing at the local grocer, Friday, July 19, 2002.

• • •

Tale by the Sea

I am usually able to walk the boardwalk at a pretty good clip. An old guy walks regularly with headsets. He warns me, "There's a speed limit along here." One day I smiled, transferred his headsets onto my head, and steered him into a fox trot. At first he was flustered. Now he looks forward to it.

Tuesday, August 13, 2002

Good Afternoon:

This morning's office visit was a treat. Thanks. Our meeting on May 28 tickled me, too. Magnificent CT scan reports move us both to the top of the class. One of us deserves a pay raise. Is it you or me?

I noticed you scratching your head in my presence. Is this why you are bald? All oncologists should be bald without choice, like their patients. Go ahead, scratch your head. Come to think of it, I see a whole string of learned practitioners following along behind me, scratching their heads, wondering, "What's up with this woman? She should be good and dead by now. We cannot find her in the medical textbooks. There is no scientific reason for her well-being."

I like the thought of balding, perplexed professionals, and I like the thought of throwing medical practices into tailspins.

Is Arimidex prolonging my existence—the drug predicted to do absolutely nothing for ER/PR negative ladies? Is my natural plan preserving me—vitamin regimen, herbal tonics, ginger, green tea, walking at the beach, deep breathing, and such? Is it God's own doing alone—his answer to a multitude of prayers?

Speaking of Arimidex, when did we last go over drug side effects? I've collected a few more. Plus, because it is my style, I make up my own. AstraZeneca's terminology for side effects is *adverse events.* Clever. Please note and record all my *adverse events* below. If I cannot decipher medical terminology, I regard it as a problem. Do you like that positive attitude? You've got to give me an A+ for effort and look at all my medical terminology!

My body as a whole experiences asthenia, back pain, headache, abdominal pain, flu syndrome, and chest pain. The digestive system fights constipation, dyspepsia, and gastrointestinal disorder. My lymphatic system complains of lymphadema. Metabolic and nutritional notations are weight gain and hypercholesteremia. The musculoskeletal region suffers arthritis, arthralgia, osteoporosis, bone pain, and arthrosis. My nervous system wrestles with depression, insomnia, dizziness, anxiety, and paraesthesia, whatever the heck that is. I complain of breast pain, (especially the one that no longer exists). Skin and appendages sweat, flash hot, and present an occasional rash. The respiratory system deals with pharyngitis, increased cough, and dyspnea. My urogenitals grumble about leukorrhea, and vulvovaginitis.

AstraZeneca omits critical urogenital adverse events, which rank high on my list of complaints; therefore, I report them for the benefit of other Arimidex patients. Additional urogenital adverse events are extinct libido, dead genitals, and burning intercourse.

Despite numerous side effects, Arimidex may be my lifeline and I will accept dead genitals over a dead body any day. Leave it to you to question, "If your genitals are dead, how do you know intercourse burns?" Silly man, out of a long list, why do you zero in on that? I refuse to answer on the grounds it may incriminate me.

Regarding my unexplained life elongation and unique drug complications, you say it best. "You and I are in the middle of a book that is not yet written."

I see you again October 1. We will add a few chapters.

Signed:

Connie

Mrs. Connie Titus
Adverse Event Specialist

• • •

Tale by the Sea

Neal pencils in *mean and vindictive* to Arimidex side effects. For example, they are constructing a condominium right across the street from my beach boardwalk. God have mercy. If anyone asks you, Connie Titus is absolutely against growth and change. My clean air, peace, restoration, and promise are drowned out by diesel fuel, noisy backhoes, cranes, concrete trucks backing and beeping, and men in hard hats yelling and pounding. Forget deep breathing. I could die from it. Friday, at my breaking point, I stomped into the sales portable to express my anger. A lady draped in black and gold and drenched with makeup said she was sincerely sorry. Yeah. I bet. She could care less, but I felt better.

Thursday, October 3, 2002

Doctor, Sir:

Well, you request to know, in detail, everything new that happens to my body, so let's go over this again.

Tuesday we read results from the MRI of my head. No malignancy shows, for which I am grateful, yet my head keeps going thump and sizzle in the night, at noontime, dawn, dusk, and during my afternoon nap. Darn it. What the heck is wrong?

The sensations started last month out of the blue. Random pains shoot through my head, not associated with headaches. There seems to be no pattern. They are not caused by, nor can I repeat them during sharp turns, bending over, or any certain movements, positions, or activities. I don't get them when a handsome man passes by, when arguing with my son about the weed-whacking, or when my sister runs ten minutes late for lunch—so they have nothing to do with sensuality, frustration, or tardiness. They happen all over the scalp, no favorite place. I will be walking along, minding my own business, and *zap*, an electrical charge shoots through my head. Some pains stop me dead on the boardwalk; others are subtle and no one knows. But I know.

Another symptom or sensation independent of the shooting pains is tingling. It starts at the top of the scalp, moves down onto my face and into my neck. What an eerie feeling and strong, too. I wonder if it is noticeable to those standing nearby—if they can see it or feel it for themselves.

A third complaint is a very sore scalp. The pain is mostly concentrated on the top of my scalp; however, I can press on a variety of spots, different each time, with localized pain. One day I could not even bear to drive with my car window down. The wind was too painful for my head. Neal took me out to eat the other night and said something unusual. I raised my eyebrows and—man! I thought my skull was going to split in half.

Some days are worse than others. I can have anywhere from three to fifteen shooting pains in one day. Tingling doesn't happen every day. Scalp soreness varies in degree but pretty much sticks around all the time. Other subtle yet annoying symptoms include memory loss, confusion, and lack of concentration. Who is on first, you or me?

Doctor, what is happening to my head?

I try not to be obsessed with cancer, but...after years of oncology, you must know if cancer survivors strain a muscle, they convince themselves it's really bone cancer and they have three to six months to live. What could this be in my head if it is not cancerous? Do you remember that unidentifiable lesion in the right frontal lobe? Is it crying out to be noticed? Is it growing and pressing on important tissue? There's been no change in hair-care products or diet lately. Neal thinks my strange post-cancer personality, behavioral changes, and ruminations are being rejected by my brain, therefore the pain. Isn't he a sweetheart?

Consider this an extra report for my chart, not the citrus box. I don't believe I am making this up, but this is one time you can honestly say it is all in my head. Please note I did not experience any of this prior to September.

When you're not doing anything (right!), please research this strange phenomenon. And the next time I complain, try not to look at me like I have two heads.

Thank you.
Over and out.

Connie

Connie

Tuesday, December 10, 2002

Alan S. Collin, M.D.:

Can I influence your practice one step further? I urge you and your partners to view a fifteen-minute video entitled *Nicole Johnson Live: Stepping into the Ring*.[41] Get ready for potent insight that will enhance your relationship with one-breasted women. I left the video on your desk.

Saturday I gathered with a scant sixteen thousand women at the TD Waterhouse Center in Orlando for a Women of Faith (WOF) Conference. It was my first WOF seminar and knew not what to expect. Nicole Johnson's dramatic portrayal of stepping into the boxing ring with breast cancer astounded me. Surely Ms. Johnson studied my personal diary in preparation. My private fearful thoughts were exposed over the loudspeaker, and I have to say it was a relief. I sobbed freely. My daughter and close friends seated next to me, at long last, knew all the specifics of my bleeding heart.

The video is short. You can do it. If you wish to order *Stepping into the Ring* for the chemo rooms or for certain patients, you can do so on the following websites: www.freshbrewedlife.com or www.womenoffaith.com or www.amazon.com. Thanks for coaching all the one-breasted ladies in the ring.

Connie

Tuesday, January 21, 2003

Dr. Collin:

This is the question of the hour: Why do you poke at my zucchini bread?

Two months ago you and Dr. Cappelletti assisted me with insurance troubles, and so, with appreciation, I presented you both with warm home-baked zucchini nut bread. Dr. Cappelletti loved it and thanked me. But a little birdie told me you stood over the bread, poked at it like a kid, and asked the entire staff if anyone had made Connie Titus mad. Yes, there are tiny green things in zucchini nut bread. Cappelletti considered it healthy. You became skeptical, thinking I might be trying to poison you. *Humphff.*

I see how you are. Golly. Live a little. Try new things.

Both you and Cappelletti recently moved your practices into new office space. For Cappelletti's new office celebration, because he trusts me, my mother-in-law and I took him and his staff a picnic basket full of homemade chicken salad, fresh breads and vegetables, and a picture-perfect, home-baked peanut butter pie (Neal's Mom's specialty).

Due to your suspicious reception of my zucchini bread, I lowered the standard for your new office celebration: enclosed is a dull, impersonal gift certificate to Garrison's Grille and a platter of boring home-baked Tollhouse cookies.

Now, don't you feel cheated? And don't you feel bad for short-changing your devoted staff?

I love you anyway,

Connie

Connie

P.S. Marissa told me how you carried the citrus box of my letters and cards over to the new office by yourself. An image of love and adoration comes to mind. I guess you love me even though I tried to poison you with zucchini nut bread, huh?

• • •

Tale by the Sea

Do you know what a hornpipe dance is? I didn't either, but I looked it up in the dictionary. A hornpipe is a lively dance formerly popular with sailors. So I am headed out to sailor or seamen property to hornpipe. If I hear any complaints, I'll give them your phone number.

Thursday, March 6, 2003

Happy Birthday, Man-Doctor,

May I offer thoughtful reflections about a child born—Alan S. Collin, M.D.?

Reflection No. 1:

Japan, April 1995— Earth, Wind & Fire appear live in concert. They present themselves on stage with a gyrating introduction to one of their best-loved classics, "That's The Way of the World." "Here we go, here we go! Clap your hands like this, yeah. Walk about. Whoa…yeah! Keep on movin', keep on groovin', keep on lovin', keep on believin'. Aah, aah, aah, owwwww!"[42]

What is the purpose of a gyrating intro? To rev up the audience. What is Earth, Wind & Fire's particular theme by doing so? "Watch me. Do as I do. Ain't life grand?" How does this correlate with the birthday of a fifty-three-year-old oncologist? I am reminded of your life's work and the potency you inject into survivorship. You go through these very motions in the chemo room on Tuesdays, like some crazy line-dance instructor. And in case you haven't noticed—your patients love it.

Reflection No. 2:

God expends concentrated effort on each individual's creation. He matches birthdates with personality and vice versa. I can just imagine our Lord's elimination process concerning your entrance into this world.

Months ending in "ary" such as January and February are for passive fence sitters, which we both know you are not. April, May, and June are proper birthdates for women. God had your mother in mind and saved her from giving birth to you in the dog days of summer. The "brrr" months of September, October, November, and December are when trees strip bare, flowers turn brown, and the earth shivers.

Elohim, another name for God as Creator, chose March as your birth month. March is a movement of steady advancement with heads held high. Warmth, wind, creativity, new beginnings, sensitivity, and a slight bit of the unusual take shape in March. All this describes your character, Alan S. Collin, M.D.

I was born in March, too. Not only are you and I Tuesday people, we are March people. That's how I recognize you, identify with you. You stand out in a crowd, like a limousine at a basketball game. (A favorite story: you taking a limousine, by yourself, to your son's basketball game. Were you wearing argyle socks?)

• • •

Oh, Happy Day—March 6, 1950. A child is born.
A child who grows into a man/instructor,
keeping us movin', groovin', lovin', believin'.
Whoa…yeah!
Celebrate. And stay young at heart, dear man!

Love from a Tuesday March kind of friend,

Connie

Connie

Tuesday, April 15, 2003

Happy Tuesday Afternoon,

Recent complaints make good sense now. A large mass that slightly relocates the vocal box will produce these things in a person:

1. Left arm numb and tingly while I sleep on my right side
2. Croaky voice
3. Chest pressure when Neal lays his body on top of mine [Smile]
4. Sandwiches go down like painful boulders

You are a hoot asking why I eat sandwiches while my husband lies on top of me. Is there any moment, any situation when a man does not think of sex? Pay attention, sir.

Do you remember why I called for scans two weeks ago? The shooting pains I've complained about in my head stepped up a notch, and I feared metastasis to my brain. We started with an MRI of the brain. You phoned me on a Friday with clear MRI results.

Next on the docket: a thyroid Doppler and neck/chest MRI. "Oops, we have a problem." CT scans, a PET scan, more detailed thyroid studies—all confirmed a large mass in the upper left mediastinum with a few solid lesions in the left lobe of the thyroid. Yet this is still not the cause of random shooting pains in my head, tingling down my face, and sore scalp because pain radiates down, not up. By the way, please, no love pats on top of my head. It hurts.

Shooting pains stepping up a notch were unmistakable signals from my body's Creator. He was nudging me to seek medical attention. I get it now, and this makes good sense.

In the spring of 2002, I commented on the fact that my drug side effects were greatly relieved after ordering Arimidex from a foreign country, at half-price, and we laughed about the possibility I was swallowing sugar pills. Hmmm. A recurrence. Sugar pills. Well, this makes good sense, too. Although I have to say, to be clean for five years and six days on a teeny, tiny white pill predicted to do absolutely nothing for me is pretty darn good, wouldn't you say?

Neal and I met with a completely new and unfamiliar doctor named Salvatore Granato, Thoracic Surgeon. The mass is inoperable, but a sliver biopsy must be obtained to aid in treatment planning. At the end of our visit, Dr. Granato said, "You know, typically, a woman with your medical history would survive only six months." Thanks. Must I hear this at every turn?

The sliver biopsy is complete. Pathology is in our hands. Inflammatory Breast Carcinoma knocks at my door a fourth time.

Again we traveled down to see our buddy Dr. Channon. Dr. Channon has mellowed through the years. Anyway, he defied the ER/PR negative theory and sent old pathology slides to Bueller University in Dallas. And he proposed other options like Fish Assay and a C-Kit test. If the C-Kit is positive, a blood factor of the tumor would respond to a new miracle drug called Gleevec, yet I find neither you nor Channon have administered this drug. That's out. I refuse to be first up to bat. With all due respect, Channon's Fish Assay, C-Kit, and Gleevec recommendations do *not* make good sense.

Neal and I also met with my radiation oncologist, Dr. R. K. With his trusty drawing board, he drew an understandable diagram of the new IRMT treatment and seemed very excited about the proposal even though I've already been zapped in that area. Dr. R. K. was the first to suggest a Lumbar Puncture (LP) to determine the cause of the shooting pains in the head. He thinks, and it makes good sense to me, the inflamed cancer cells may be collecting in the lining of the brain and would not highlight on CT scans or an MRI. I will agree to the LP, but decline IRMT.

Oh, God. What is wrong with my body? I wobble, flimsy

and useless. Why is my canvas scarred and weakened with ugly spots? My tent is no longer strong or secure. I am officially frightened now. I am the little tent dweller starring in the poem below.

O, Mr. Tentmaker

It was nice living in this tent when it was strong and secure, and the sun was shining and the air was warm. But, Mr. Tentmaker, it's scary now. You see, my tent is acting like it is not going to hold together. The poles seem weak and they shift with the wind. A couple of stakes have wiggled loose from the sand; and worst of all, the canvas has a rip. It no longer protects me from beating rain or stinging fly. It's scary in here, Mr. Tentmaker.

Last week I went to the repair shop and some repairman tried to patch the rip in my canvas. It didn't help much, though, because the patch pulled away from the edges and now the tear is worse. What troubled me most, Mr. Tentmaker, is that the repairman didn't even seem to notice that I was still in the tent. He just worked on the canvas while I shivered inside. I cried out once, but no one heard me.

I guess my first real question is: Why did you give me such a flimsy tent? I can see by looking around the campground that some of the tents are much stronger and more stable than mine. Why, Mr. Tentmaker, did you pick a tent of such poor quality for me? And even more important, what do you intend to do about it?

• • •

O, little tent dweller, as the Creator and Provider of tents, I know all about you and your tent, and I love you both. I made a tent for myself once and lived in it on your campground. My tent was vulnerable, too, and some vicious attackers ripped it to pieces, while I was still in it.

It was a terrible experience, but you will be glad to know they couldn't hurt me; in fact, the whole occurrence was a tremendous advantage because it is this very victory over my enemy that frees me to be a present help to you.

O, little tent dweller, I am now prepared to come and live in your tent with you, if you will invite me. You'll learn as we dwell together that real security comes from my being in your tent with you. When the storms come, you can huddle in my arms, and I'll hold you. When the canvas rips, we'll go to the repair shop together.

Some day, little tent dweller, some day your tent is going to collapse; you see, I've designed it only for temporary use. But when it does, you and I are going to leave together. I promise not to leave before you do. And then, free of all that would hinder or restrict, we will move to our permanent home and together, forever, we will rejoice and be glad. [43]

• • •

"Therefore we do not lose heart. Though outwardly we are wasting away, yet inwardly we are being renewed day by day" (2 Corinthians 4:16, NIV). Gee whiz. When I am settled into fear and wasting away, some well-meaning friend slips me a note straight from God himself, forcing my shoulders to relax. Don't you just hate it when that happens?

The reparation/renewal plan with you, good man, is a little Navelbine, with no hair loss, and a little Xeloda, with no hair loss. Sounds like a plan. I stand up, straighten my spine, and relax the shoulders. Let us start. Where do I sign?

With my hand in your hand, you ushered me to the Tuesday morning chemo room and sat me down in the company of Jane Valentino, Dorothy Lunsford, and Danielle Tilton. I was about to rub elbows with miraculous, surviving, spiritual heroes in the arena of life. This too, made good sense.

Love,

Connie

Connie Titus, a flimsy, torn tent dweller

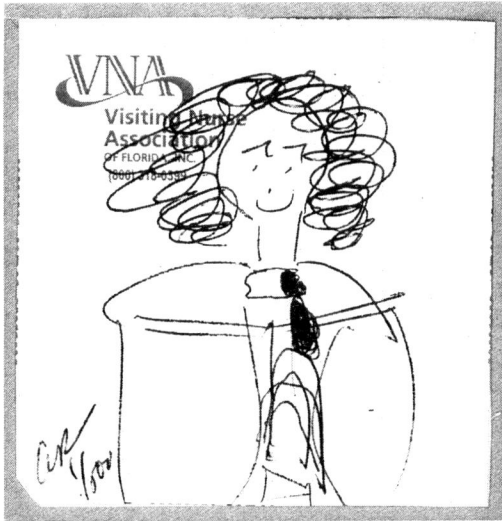

Dr. Collin's personal artwork of fourth recurrence—new tumors. Doctor portrayed Patient as a faceless, hairless figure. In order to save face, patient penciled in her important features.

Wednesday, July 16, 2003—2:43 a.m.

My Dear Physician:

Notice the time this letter is written. Low-dose steroids slipped into my pre-drug mix turn me into a hyper insomniac superwoman. There is no sleeping on treatment night. Ever. Neal and I count on it. You say such a small dose cannot prevent me from sleeping. Ha. You're funny.

Steroids are good—steroids are bad. On the good side, my mind is clear. The middle of the night offers quiet time to decipher, organize, pay bills and balance, correspond, remember everything I previously forgot, and write lists of things to do. Energy surges are exciting but most often resisted. If my family and neighborhood were not sleeping, I would run the vacuum, re-arrange the furniture, and build on an addition to the house. No, I am not out for hire.

My family says steroids are bad because while I sleep the next day, they are stuck with endless lists of chores. Steroids are bad for me because if I go with the incredible physical power, my back is thrown out of whack. The other bad news is the crash from high energy into the low sensations listed below.

Tell me again why we do steroids—to pad the effects of chemotherapy drugs? I don't understand.

Disease and chemicals wrestle inside my body, which shoves me into a state of suspense. Am I going to die now or not? Tell me. Every clinic or diagnostic center I enter, every physician I come in contact with insinuates I am a dead-woman walking. Some days (or nights) I accept the title with pride and march ahead strong. Other days a picture of me as a dead-woman walking bars the doors and shuts down the system.

The idea of recurrence came to me last September, long before red flags jumped off reports in March. So I've had a little private time to get used to the idea. Still, the final decree and reality jolt me.

Yesterday, while waiting for you to grace me with your presence, I read your office notes from last week's visit. It is your opinion that Navelbine and Xeloda cause me slight discomfort. You state my treatment is well tolerated. What? I was not strong enough to argue with you in person, but I have no problem arguing on paper. See my rebuttal below and hear me shouting!

Flu-like symptoms, body aches, headaches, weakness, and fatigue consume me. Food and water taste metallic. Light duty causes me to huff and puff like a ninety-year-old. I don't care to talk, write, listen to music, watch TV, sleep, sit, stand, swim, or walk. That means I will not, under any circumstance, dance at daybreak. And I no longer apologize for haughty temperament. My body bloats. The apparel of choice is big, man-sized shirts with no brassiere. I suffer chest pains and simulated heart attacks on a regular basis.

You recently went to bed for five days with flu-like symptoms, body aches, headaches, weakness, and fatigue. Was that *slight* discomfort for you?

Flipping again to a positive, those three women you introduced me to, Dorothy, Jane, and Danielle, gosh—thanks. There's a whole lot of learnin' and lovin' going on in your chemo room, not to mention the light that comes bursting in. I try to schedule my appointments near theirs. Dorothy's earthly news may not be too hopeful, yet she carries herself with the joy of our Lord. Her divine purpose and mission shine wherever she is. Jane, we call her Queen Jane, tackles the unknown with humor. There's no other way for her to cope. Danielle's eyes light up when she talks about her work at the bank, and from where I sit, I can almost hear her white cells multiplying. Each gal makes the following passage a reality:

> When darkness overtakes him, light will come bursting in … Such a man will not be overthrown by evil circumstances. God's constant care of him will make a deep

impression on all who see it. He does not fear bad news, nor live in dread of what may happen. For he is settled in his mind that Jehovah will take care of him.

Psalm 112:4, 6-7 (TLB)

Dorothy, Jane, and Danielle tolerate their conditions and refuse to be overthrown by evil circumstances. I want to be like them, but how?

On another subject, you've heard me refer to you as my cutest, most cuddly teddy bear, and this is the reason why I love you so much. Well, on occasion, you prove yourself less than cuddly or cute—but, since I am abnormal, I love you even more during these episodes.

Midstream in our office visit yesterday, Marissa knocked on the door, summoning you to a phone call. Instead of taking it back in your office, you talked on the phone in the hallway, right outside my door. I knew right away whom you were talking to. Your fever and pitch broke the thermometer, turning you into a stark, raving lunatic. The phone slammed onto the hook while the person on the other end (your mother) was still talking. You bolted back into my cubicle, shaking your head, apologizing. "I'm sorry. She is the only one who can turn me into an unruly child!"

Last night Neal and I conducted a family meeting with our teenage son, his girlfriend, and a troubled friend of theirs who has been camping out with us. I spoke my mind. My son's fever and pitch also broke all sound barriers until he turned into a stark, raving lunatic, a carbon copy of you earlier. The candle on the table extinguished. Mommies do somehow bring out the worst in their sons. I blame chemo and steroids. Is your mom on chemo?

With love, still, even when I say phooey on you!

Connie

Connie

Tuesday, July 22, 2003

Hello to He Who Wears a Bright Blue Dress Shirt:

Do you realize you've looked at my chest wall more often in six years of practice than my husband has in thirty-three years of marriage? He better get on the ball.

After your usual look/see in the cubicle, I sauntered toward the chemo room for blood work and a treatment. My white counts were too low, though, and Nurse Nicole summoned you into the nurse's station to confer. You hollered out to me, "Connie, you suffer bone pain with Neulasta or Neupogen shots, right?"

"Right!" I agreed quickly and added loud enough for all to hear, "You would have to handcuff me and chase me down the hallway in order to give me one of those shots."

Oohs and *aahs* broke out in the chemo room.

Peeking out the door wearing a slight blush and wide grin, you commented, "That sounds like an intriguing man-woman type of game."

Louder *oohs* and *aahs* and some applause arose from the chemo patrons. You then admonished me, "Shhh. Now these people know what we do together."

I stood up from my reclining chair and walked towards you to define the substitute ingredients for my white-cell elevation. Chemo patient ears flipped in our direction so I whispered.

First, your bright blue long-sleeve shirt alone brings white cells into normal range. Next, I prescribed for myself a close embrace—close enough to soak up some of your time-released aftershave. White blood cells will then rise to 10.0 or higher. Yes, a blue, scented embrace holds twice the power of any drug and makes me good to go, especially if I can take a week's vacation from your pesky chemo.

The blue, scented embrace was conducted to the sound of more applause.

Today I decided to stick around a while longer. Away with last week's dead-woman walking. I am alive and well and ready for a shindig.

My adoration for you exceeds the recommended daily allowance. Shall we report this to the FDA or will it be our secret?

Connie

Connie, smiling

Saturday, September 20, 2003

Dear Friend:

My large mass—where is it? It is gone, disappeared into thin air. Hip, hip, hooray for Navelbine and prayer and Xeloda and prayer. Malignancy conquered in such a short time. Seriously, have you ever seen anything like this before? God has unlimited miracles up his sleeve for me. Thanks for assisting him, Dr. Collin.

May I share a Messianic story that relates to my husband? I know. Doctors do not have time for this sort of nonsense, but I think I am supposed to offer you a few more prescriptions. Plus, there's something about you that makes me want to share every single facet of my living. Are you still with me?

Once upon a time, the Master/Teacher was partaking of a meal with his friends for the very last time. Midway through the evening, he got up from the table, took off his robe, wrapped a towel around his groin, and began gently washing his disciples' feet. Some of them protested. They argued that a gesture such as this was below him. He kept on with his offering of friendship for each and every one of them, never questioning their love or devotion for him. These quiet moments of courtesy were not contingent on man's past or future behavior. It's what I call true love.

I am a member of a small group Bible study. My friends and I discussed the main reason for Christ washing the disciples' feet. Was it strictly the cultural custom of hygiene of that time or a washing away of their sins? Was it a good deed Jesus wished his friends would pass along or was it his authority in action (I'll do what I want to, when I want to, whether you want me to, or not)? Is it our lesson on humble servitude today—Jesus' command to love one another? I believe it was merely his response to their friendship. He was filled with love from deep within his heart. The Bible clearly states, "And how he loved his disciples!" (John 13:3b, TLB). Love one another. Love is the answer.

While reading this story over and over again, I remembered a time when Christ washed my feet. Actually it was my Christ-like husband. That good man named Jesus has taken up residence inside the man I live with.

One evening after my mastectomy, Neal helped me disrobe and step into the bathtub of warm water. There I sat, literally cut in half, bloated, with two ugly blood-filled drains sprouting from my side. He tenderly bathed his unrecognizable bride, smiled with his eyes, and whispered how beautiful I was to him…as if nothing in his world had ever changed. Love one another. Love is the answer.

There have been numerous washing-of-feet episodes in this household since. On nights of discomfort, or insomnia, or untimely excretion of bodily fluids due to flu-bugs or chemical reactions, I remove myself from our marriage suite to retire at the other end of the house. Neal must arise somewhat refreshed and go to work each day, whether I am wrestling with disease or not. But his loving attention never sleeps. When he rolls over and notices I'm not beside him, this is what happens: My devoted husband stumbles and/or gropes through a pitch-black house without his glasses or his teeth, wearing nothing but his Fruit of the Loom boxer briefs, just so he can touch his beloved bride's cheek for fever, offer me a cool or warm drink, an ice pack or a heating pad, a foot massage, or simply a word of kindness in the dark.

Tears well up as I write this. Neal is so full of love for lopsided me. Love is the answer.

Listen to England Dan and John Ford Coley's lyrics to "Love Is the Answer":

> …I can't stay here any more…who knows why, someday we all must die. It's a lonely, lonely world—people turn their heads, and walk on by. Tell me is it worth just another try?…And when you feel afraid (love one another.) And

when you've lost your way (love one another.) And when you're all alone (love one another.) And when you're far from home (love one another.) And when you're down and out (love one another.) And when your hope's run out (love one another.) And when you're near the end—love—we've got to love—we've got to love one another. Chorus: Light of the world, shine on me, love is the answer. Shine on us all, set us free, love is the answer. [44]

The idea of loving one another in all situations sustains survivorship. I withdraw to nature, the ocean side, for prayer. "O God, Light of the World, shine on me, love is the answer. Thank you, Matchmaker, for teaming me up with a noble gentleman named Neal. He doesn't turn his head, he doesn't walk on by, he doesn't say he can't stay here any more. When I feel afraid, when I've lost my way, when I'm down and out, or my hope has run out, he comes to me gently, in the dark, with love. Love is the answer. Thank you, dear God. I worship your Holy Name. Amen."

Dr. Collin, I give thanks, too, for the way you love patients when their hope runs out. I saw you on your knees in the chemo room the other day, talking softly with our former Mayor. His hope was running out. Your compassion fills in the gaps for all of us.

Connie

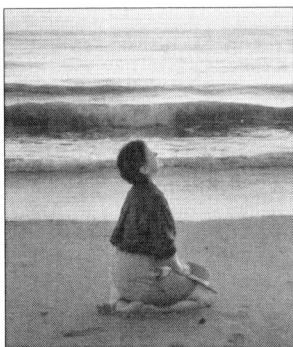

Patient Connie prays to God the Father beachside. "...a profound tie exists between the health of the soul and the health of the body... our bodies have their best chance for health when our spiritual lives are healthy" (J. Ellsworth Kalas, The Grand Sweep, p. 33).

Courtesy of Photographer Nina Jackes

Wednesday, November 26, 2003

Alan S. Collin, M.D.,

Seasons come and go by appointment of our most Gracious God. *Thou hast brought us through the circuit of another bountiful harvest (and successful chemo regimen).*

Under the influence of your cubicle winks, whistling, and fancy dance steps, my white cells multiplied and made it possible for Neal and my cancer-free body to take a colorful excursion to our homeland. Golden lights and soft shadows urged me into a Scotch/Irish jig in Central Ohio. After that, I sought a quiet place to give thanks and your name came up.

I suppose every creature on earth is a survivor of something or other. From dawn to dusk people should acknowledge the sanctity of life.

Tomorrow Americans will gather with families and friends around tables—holding hands and formally bowing in reverence to God Eternal. We are ever mindful of the hopes of life, the powers of mind and body, peaceful homes where freedom rings, a bountiful harvest, endless love and compassion, and friends who stand steady—blessings that make this business of surviving the best it can be.

'Tis the season to personally honor you, sir.

Thank you for teaching me how to behold meaningful moments of beauty and laughter...one right after another.

All my life I've yearned for the protection and teasing of a big brother. Tag, you're it, you fit the design.

You navigate my husband and me through uncharted waters. You share in the mysterious miracle(s) of my body. With appreciation, we believe in you.

Thank you for serving, in person, homemade fudge to needy patients in your chemo room, then having enough sense to run for your life. It is a proven fact that within twenty minutes, chocolate makes me mean. Mr. Titus says I grow horns.

I am grateful for that light, bright, spacious chemo room at 2100 Nottingham Avenue where miracle gals assemble on Tuesday mornings. A certain degree of merriment erupts. We celebrate the common cord who binds us together, God Almighty, and we're delighted he elected you our professor of merriment.

Thanks for handling me as if I am whole and hopeful.

Admitting you don't know, when you truly, simply, do not know, kindles great respect in my heart. Bless your human-ness.

I like the way you and I easily interchange our titles of Team Captain, Team Player, Cheerleader, and Locker-Room Monitor. To my knowledge, neither one of us has yet to get the upper hand.

Thanks for teaching us all a valuable lesson by way of codeine overdose. ("Do as I say, not as I do!" a common, comical practice among physicians.)

Thank you for allowing me to meet your bride this year. Getting together with Jeanne for giggles and whispers increased my adoration for you.

Yesterday I whipped out my personal stethoscope for cross-examination. I also inquired whether or not you are capable of stopping for a gallon of milk on the way home from work. Malignant eruptions in a human body give permission for unconventional behavior or speech, and I take full advantage of the privilege. You may not know what to expect from me, but you always play along. That, my good man, is devotion.

Alan S. Collin, M.D., you never fail to do the good that lies next to your hand. Your life's work is your testimony. The God of creation can fix things all by himself, but he chooses to work through people. Thanks for answering his call.

May there be much triumphant rejoicing in the Collin household this Thanksgiving.

Forever your friend,

Connie

Connie

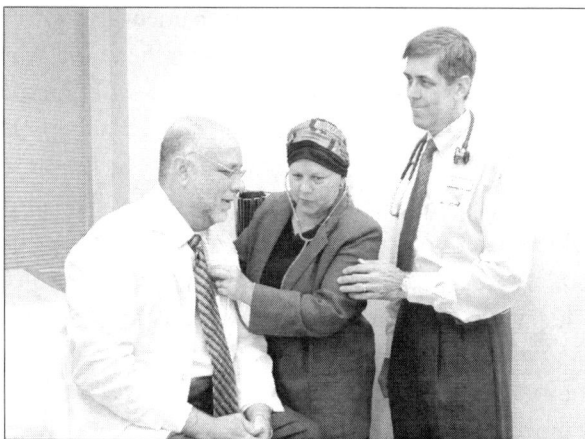

Office visit role reversal. Directed by Physician Assistant Steve Riley, Patient Connie monitors Dr. Collin's heart rate and respiration.

Courtesy of Photographer Jerry Brewer

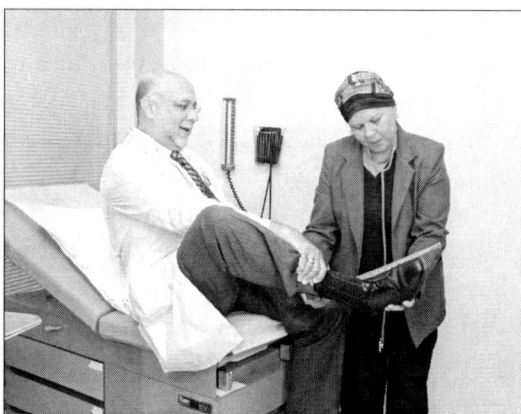

Patient measures Doctor's shoe size because all is fair in cross-examination.

Courtesy of Photographer Jerry Brewer

Tuesday, January 27, 2004

My Doctor:

Today is my seventh mastectomy anniversary. Thanks for a positively good check-up.

Last week our daughter convinced me to get a tattoo on my scar line. She saw an exciting presentation on the Discovery channel. Breast cancer survivors are dressing up their mastectomies with unique tattoos. My little girl has a way of jump-starting me when I am stalled in life, so I listen, no matter the subject line. Tattoos are totally out of character for me and forbidden in this household. I feel the fad is a gross dishonor of God's workmanship. So both God and my husband were dumbfounded to think I would even consider tainting my body in such a way.

Daydreaming kicked in, though, and drew me up the perfect emblem. By cutting off my left breast, my beating heart is exposed and even drops out on occasion. And when I stumble through dramatic treatment, my dropped-out, beating heart is held in the strong hands of authorities—my husband, my doctor, my God. That's my perfect emblem. A beating heart held by two strong, authoritative hands.

The first two doctors who listened to this tattoo idea shouted, "Risk, danger, insanity, sheer stupidity!" I wondered if you would be receptive to this idea and was anxious to hear what your humorous response would consist of. But I didn't even approach the subject. The idea was put to rest before I entered your presence. Here is the reason.

While back in the chemo room for blood work, I spied a new book on the shelf. *Art.Rage.Us.*[45] is a collection of art, photography, and literary work by breast-cancer survivors. This is a startling, graphic picture book. Pain-filled expressions by carved-upon spirits fill large pages. Some of these women are badly scarred.

My mind and body traveled back in time to 1997 when healthcare professionals looked at my mastectomy for the first time. I got the same response across the board: big smiles of amazement and comments about how my surgeon, Marvin J. Cappelletti, M.D., did a good job on me. I smiled too, mildly impressed. But the magnitude did not register. I never considered the vantage point from which these professionals speak. Perhaps it is good manners toward all mastectomy patients to build their self-esteem. Curiosity never led me to approach other lopsided women with the invitation, "I'll show you mine if you show me yours." All this time I've had nothing to compare myself to…until now.

Horror shots of other mastectomies in this book sobered me, and I beheld a new appreciation of my beautiful, smooth, easy-on-the-eye scar line. Who needs a tattoo? I am already unique.

On my way home, I stopped by Dr. Marvin J. Cappelletti's office to hug his neck, kiss him, and thank him for the skill of his hand and expertise of his practice—with no regard for the fact that Dr. Marvin J. Cappelletti hates hugging and kissing. [Smile]

One more thing, then you should get back to work. Driving over to the beach the other day, I noticed something. Remember when I reported Arimidex deadens a woman's genitals? After being away from the drug for a while, I am now pleased to report vibrations while driving a vehicle. It is awake down there.

With that boyish grin and pen in hand, you asked to record the make and model of my vehicle(s) and the route/roads traveled. Is this an entry for the revised medical text you are writing or a personal note to slip in your shirt pocket for Jeanne? Okay. Here you go.

Titus vehicles: 1996 Silver/Teal Dodge Ram pickup truck; 2002 Dark Green Malibu 4-door sedan.

Roads traveled: Tangelo Avenue Extension to Southwest Federation Highway; North to Seaside Drive and the beach or South to Mr. Titus' place of business where he is willing to put out any fires. [Bigger Smile]

The vibration story would make a cute entry for the book *Art.Rage.Us.* Next time you walk a patient back to the chemo room, ask Nurse Nicole to show you this book I speak of. It's not entirely jagged edges. There are some fun themes. Pages 67, 90, and 167 are my favorites.

Thanks for holding my beating heart in your hands. Thanks for your interest in vehicular vibrations.

Signed,

Connie

Connie—Ms. Tattoo-less (not Ms. Tight Ass, as some people mispronounce Titus). Oh, you may also address me as Ms. Port-less. A six-year relationship with a foreign object inside my chest wall ended in December. The infusaport became inflamed and Cappelletti took it out. He dug it out, tugged and sawed and ripped for hours on end. I cannot, for the life of me, understand why surgeons install infusaports with anesthesia in the hospital but remove them with the patient fully awake in the doctor's office. I am a little nervous without a port. What if I need treatments by infusion again?

Tuesday, March 2, 2004

Happy Birthday, My Fifty-Four-Year-Old Musical Medicine Man:

Celebrate with three dozen melodies. Music is the best gift—one of God's greatest inventions. Follow instructions.

Gift No. 1: Diana Krall's voice reminds Neal of Peggy Lee. Our daughter says Diana's CD *When I Look in Your Eyes* is good medicine after a long, hard day. Do oncologists have an occasional long, hard day? Duh. Here is your medicine. Unravel yourself. You are to plop down in your easy chair, turn the lights down low, and open a bottle of fine wine because Robert Louis Stevenson claims, "Wine is bottled poetry."[46]

Leslie Bricusse wrote the lyrics to "When I Look in Your Eyes." Do you know this person? Is Leslie your patient? I ask because this song describes your eyes *exactly* as I see them. Included are the stars, the importance of the sea, and the way your business works.

> When I look in your eyes, I see the wisdom of the world in your eyes; I see the sadness of a thousand goodbyes…the softness of the moon…the gentle sparkle of the stars…the deepness of the sea; I see the deepness of the love, the love I feel you feel for me; I see the passing of the years…and when we part there will be no tears, no goodbyes, I'll just look into your eyes. Those eyes, so wise, so warm, so real; how I love the world your eyes reveal.[47]

Enjoy a moving musical picture of your eyes. Sadly I must inform you—don't choke—upon research, the lyricist who describes your eyes so beautifully…is a man.

Gift No. 2: I try again to brassercise a woodwind with Canadian Brass' CD *Swingtime*. Who would have thought you to be a bassoonist when you represent all the back row, low brass qualifications known to mankind (assertive, yet soft around the edges; balding; humorous; nice full lips). I offer you another Canadian Brass recording with embellishment of rhythm, strings, and woodwinds. Let CB usher you into a smoky club back in the '50s, where Cole, Duke, Count, and Ira are very much alive. Track 11, though, is different. It almost doesn't fit. "Concierto de Aranjuez" is a sketch of a city in Spain.[48] Rarely can I listen to this number without a sudden emotional outburst. Turn up the "Concierto" to full sound and retreat once more to that easy chair in the dark. Wine is optional.

Gift No. 3: Let us go back to 1967 with Moody Blues in *Days of Future Passed.* If you were to revisit music of your youth, what would be your preference? I toyed between this and *A Decade of Steely Dan,* although I could be way off base in both cases. When you put this CD in, be patient. The first song takes a few minutes to rev up. Poetry, the beat group, and a symphony orchestra feed on each other's imagination to paint a picture of every man's day. Don't get too comfortable. Heavy metal of Track 4 might jolt you. Listen to "The Afternoon—Forever Afternoon (Tuesday?)" lyrics on Track 5.[49] I am reminded of our Tuesdays. I come home from Tuesday morning appointments with a handful of life lessons. Tuesday afternoons are spent trying to interpret them and you. The main conclusion: you definitely know how to chase dark clouds away. While listening to the Moody Blues, forget the wine. Go for hard liquor. How old were you in 1967? Old enough for hard liquor?

I bid you a gleeful day...and command you to sing...now. "Sing and make music in your heart to the Lord..." (Ephesians 5:19, NIV).

Connie

P.S. One of my big-brother daydreams is to take a road trip with you. Jeanne can still sit in the passenger seat next to you. I will sit behind you, and the three of us can harmonize the whole way there and back. We might miss a few exits.

Tuesday, August 3, 2004

Help! Dr. Collin! Help!

The airplane door flung wide open at 13,500 feet. Over water. What was I thinking?

God has a sense of humor. When our son graduated eighth grade, I promised him *if* and *when* he graduated high school, I would go skydiving with him. This was an outlandish statement for someone who throws up on commercial flights. I made the promise with the understanding I would be dead by then. Remember, at that time, I had failed all aggressive treatment. All physicians, including you, thought that if I lived six months, it would be a miracle.

Three years later I was still kicking around giving orders. Ron was to graduate in one year. I tried to downgrade my promise to parasailing, but he would have no part of it. Neal, bless his heart, thought himself helpful by finding a website for Skydive Allandale where they offer tandem skydiving. He was excited to show me photos of people actually doing this...crazy people.

> "You have to jump off cliffs all the time,
>
> and build your wings on the way down."[50]

Three months prior to graduation I came running into your office, pleading for your doctor's excuse why I must not skydive. You quickly reminded me of my two herniated discs. Well, I *had* herniated discs. They are healed, but yes, I will use that. However, your professional verbal excuse carried no weight with our son.

Dragging my feet, I got in touch with Skydive Allandale. They seemed eager to make all my *dreams* come true. I told them I must interview whoever would be strapped to my back. I would go down the line like a drill sergeant testing the strength in their legs; taking measurements; inspecting strapping gear; looking for compassionate, clear eyes and alert brain function; and asking one pertinent question, "Let us have a show of hands.

How many of you are friends with Jesus?" Once my final choice was made, I would offer my tandem instructor a list of sweet nothings to whisper in my ear on the way down.

Dr. Collin, do you believe your traditional, conventional, moderate patient-friend would even consider such bizarre action?

An interesting development: the week of graduation brought with it the beginning of a new chemo regimen. My cancer came back to haunt me. Some people, including Ron, said I would go to any great length not to skydive. Yep. That's one way to take care of it.

After four months of treatment, though, the large mass disappeared. The next ten months were cancer-free, making the pathway to Skydive Allandale clear and sunny. My family preached bravery and trust until I agreed to take my miracle and try something new. Besides, God wanted me to keep a promise to our only son.

I think we were all in agreement: *What can happen to me that isn't already looming in the wings?*

Promise fulfilled. On Sunday morning, August 1, 2004, I did it. My whole family did it. After signing a four-page what-if waiver, loading up on Dramamine, and being strapped to our assigned tandem buddies, we jumped out of a fully-fueled, all-props-operating airplane over Ponce de Leon Inlet. I chose a Sunday morning knowing our church family would be inside the chapel praying for us. I stepped out, right on top of a cloud. The view was absolutely magnificent.

Am I glad I went through with this? I think so. Would I do it again? Probably not. Would I recommend friends, such as you, jump onto a cloud at 13,500 feet? Yes, go for it. I know how much you *love* to fly. [NOT]

Building my wings on the way
down (or up),

Connie

Connie

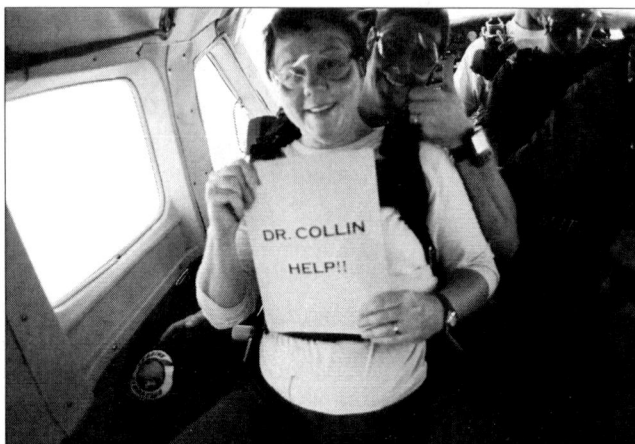

Patient Connie is about to jump out an open airplane door at 13,500 feet with a man strapped to her back. Although Connie's facial expression does not jive with the panic in her gut, she utters (by sign) one last plea to Doctor.

Courtesy of Photographer Ian Brown

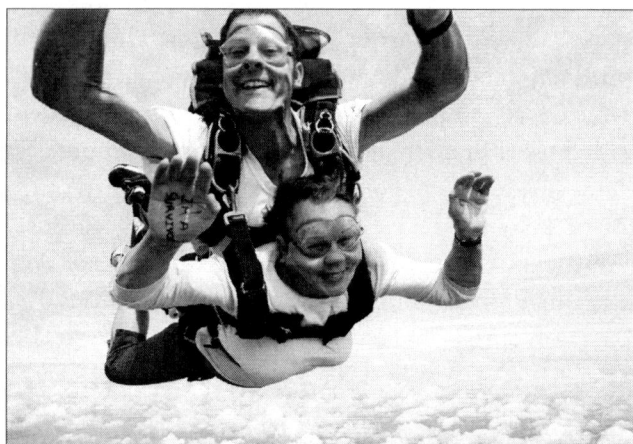

Patient Connie's actual tandem flight through mid-air—an out-of-body, never-to-be-repeated experience.

Courtesy of Photographer Ian Brown

Tuesday, August 17, 2004
(This is a business letter. Read thoroughly; do not skim).

Dr. Collin:

Don't you just want to hogtie the chick who isn't satisfied until she finds something wrong?

I take time away from the truly needy. So, after you hogtie me, will you please refer me somewhere? My symptoms are obviously not malignant. Send me to an internist, or maybe I should try neurosurgeon Bonnie Burgess again, or a shrink.

Despite clear scans, I don't feel well. I am not able to function. Head trauma (random shooting pains, tingling, very sore scalp) is worse, and since the cause cannot be found—I am at my wit's end. Now my torso has many of the same symptoms.

Wearing a brassiere is painful. Tender spots, shooting pains in the chest and rib cage are all concentrated on the left side. I am uncomfortable sleeping on my left side and tummy. I am attacked by simulated heart-attack chest pains and tightness. They are mild to moderate and very unsettling. Simple tasks cause a shortness of breath. Turtlenecks choke me. Singing hurts. The short version is that I would feel better if Cappelletti amputated at the waist.

Do I still have a clear understanding of Inflammatory Breast Carcinoma? IBC is an advanced, accelerated form of breast cancer staged as IIIB or IV. IBC is usually not detected by mammograms or ultrasounds. IBC camps out inside the lymphatic system, which is part of the immune system that protects against infection and disease. The cancer cells clog the lymphatic system just below the skin. IBC usually grows in nests or sheets rather than a confined, solid tumor; therefore, it can spread without a detectable lump. Twenty-one lymph nodes have been removed from the left axilla and twenty nodes removed from the right axilla, causing my torso to function like an automobile without an oil filter. Correct?

Every morning Neal performs a light massage therapy on both arms. That is how we keep lymphadema under control. But the fluid ends up in my armpit area and hangs out there until I move it down while bathing. Am I moving the bacteria in this lymph fluid down into the mesenteric lymph nodes? Am I causing Lymphorrhagia (escape of the lymph from the vessels?)

You are rolling your eyeballs, thinking, *Oh no, here comes her medical terminology again.*

Are CT scans and PET scans limited to tumors or masses in organs and bones? Would sheets/nests in tissues or fluid show up? I am reminded there was no alarm on my initial mammogram or ultrasound. Cappelletti could not detect from any scan that thirteen of twenty-one nodes in the left axilla and eight of twenty nodes in the right axilla were diseased until he cut in there. Are CT scans and PET scans front view only, or do they examine the body sides and back including muscles, soft tissue, spinal cord, and cervical spine? Do these scans peer inside bones, inside the brain?

What was the result of my right mammogram done March 4, 2004? Can you give me the calcium, C-reactive protein, sedimentation rate, and tumor marker scores from the blood chemistry collected March 16?

Do I need an antibiotic or an anti-inflammatory drug? Is a virus, bacteria, parasite, or fungus growing inside me? But blood work would show this, right? What about Herpes Zoster, better known as shingles? If you recall, I had multiple itching eruptions all over the torso last summer. And it was near where these tender spots are now. I've had sores on my scalp before, too. Help me out, here. Work with me, buddy. I am trying hard to diagnose myself.

Would a lymphangiography or lymphagraphy benefit me?

Will blood chemistry and/or scans detect Pachymeningitis, Lymphangiosarcoma, Lupus, Erythematosus, Lymphangitis, Astrocytoma, Lymphorrhagia, Glioblastoma, Encephalitis, Oligodendroglioma, Encephalomyelitis, Ependymoma, Hematoma, Hemangioblastoma, Meningioma, or Leptomeningitis?

Even though I claim dysfunction, I just joined a beginner line-dancing class. Do you think the women dancing on either side of me can tell I am loaded with diseases I cannot pronounce?

Am I driving you nuts, or do you want to hire me for medical transcription? But who can tell if I'm spelling these conditions correctly because the computer underlines every one of them in red. Tell me to take a hike and I will live quietly with all my obsessive-compulsive hypochondria. Contact me at the Rising Hope facility on Medallion Road, a loony bin where all women with imaginary diseases reside. Maybe they teach line-dancing.

Signed,

Connie

Obsessive-compulsive Connie

• • •

Tale by the Sea

I drag my hypochondriac body to the sea for answers. The lifeguard on duty might give me an acceptable diagnosis. The Lifeguard in the sky might give me an acceptable diagnosis, if I earnestly ask him, trusting, believing.

> But when you ask him, be sure that you really expect him to tell you, for a doubtful mind will be as unsettled as a wave of the sea that is driven and tossed by the wind; and every decision you then make will be uncertain, as you turn first this way, and then that. If you don't ask with faith, don't expect the Lord to give you any solid answer.
>
> James 1:6-8 (TLB)

Monday, October 4, 2004

To My Fellow Pisces Man-Doctor Who Regards Running Water Paramount:

I can just picture your panic. So post-hurricane, you ran helter-skelter through your house trying all the faucets?

After surviving seven and a half years of cancer and treatment and taking great measure to stay alive, forecasts of strong winds peeling away our roof and sucking me out like a vacuum sounded outrageous. Below is my A-Z commentary on this business of hurricanes:

a. Most of us still don't know what day it is.

b. I will not sit through another storm. A vibrating, shaking, rattling, and rolling house for hours on end is not for me. I would rather, gladly, jump out of an airplane.

c. Ten days without power or running water is my limit.

d. Our new roof and screened porch did marvelously well, so as soon as I find our contractors, I will make love to them in the backyard.

e. Utility men with gear and trucks leave their families and come from every corner of our United States to restore us, and I, for one, am thankful.

f. Driving around town, touring friends' homes, or what's left of them, makes me sick to my stomach.

g. Explosive diarrhea is almost a daily event. It is probably a result of living out of coolers for ten days. Diarrhea is a true adventure with no running water.

h. Whiskey with Cheetos is appropriate breakfast food during hurricanes.

i. Most folks are courteous at big intersections where traffic lights lay in pieces on the ground, but there is always one bad apple that causes tires to squeal and blood pressure to rise, resulting in motorists of all ages needing clean underwear, of which there is none.

j. Neighbors congregate morning, noon, and night to nail on tarps or scrap tarpaper in driving rain and wind. They offer eggs from a generated fridge or loan chainsaws, rakes, PVC pipe, and manpower to boot. This has to be a good thing.

k. Taking a bath in the next door neighbor's swimming pool littered with aluminum planks, timber, and shingles is not so bad—in fact, it is a relief from the heat. Hey, when it is pitch black, who can see that debris anyway? All you need is a bar of soap.

l. Families on porches, talking softly in the dark, playing board games by lantern, becoming attached at the hip are things we should have thought of long before any storm.

m. Living with a man who knows how to fix everything is a delight. And each morning he puts on his rubber hip boots, pulls his little red wagon out to the johnboat near the pasture where he collects a five-gallon bucket of water, and adds bleach to it so his family can flush one toilet, once every day. He is ingenuity at its best.

n. Clothes, books, furniture, computers, and TV's *ain't no thing* compared to living, breathing, the safety of a loved one, and finding a dry place to lay your head at night.

o. I plan to look up descendants of Thomas Edison, the inventors of A/C, automatic washing machines, and refrigerators and write them sincere thank-you notes. These things I will never again take for granted.

p. Rules relax. Bob the dog gets away with lounging on forbidden furniture while we concern ourselves with eating ice cream before it melts.

q. How many mosquito bites can a human being survive in one night?

r. Mealtime requires creativity. Pizza can be cooked on the grill (very carefully). We enjoy a picnic every day, complete with ants and flies.

s. Any family member using real silverware, plates, or cups is in big trouble with me.

t. There is no ice to be had anywhere.

u. Way worse than that, there is no ice cream to be had anywhere. For days and weeks and forever we scream for ice cream.

v. My beach. Oh, Lord my God! How or why did he turn my place of healing beauty into a battle zone? Vegetation is brown. Boardwalks are ripped up like toothpicks. Sand is piled twelve feet high. Archibald's outdoor restaurant is no more. One more time, oh, my God!

w. How does a community go about putting itself back together?

x. The elderly, the sick, and poor are without a roof over their heads. Knee-deep insulation and ceiling materials stick like mud to what little they own. The stench of rotting food inside warm refrigerators and mildewing wet linens bagged for days brings death a little too close. These folks must make life-changing decisions and fill out endless paperwork at ages eighty and ninety. Who will help them?

y. Where is God? What is he trying to tell us? Where do we go from here?

z. Singing "It Is Well with My Soul"[51] in four-part harmony with sunbeams shining through stained-glass windows of a little chapel is a great start. Let there be rebuilding and pulling together with resources. Let there be relishing of simple pleasures.

Love from a Piscean survivor,

Connie

Connie

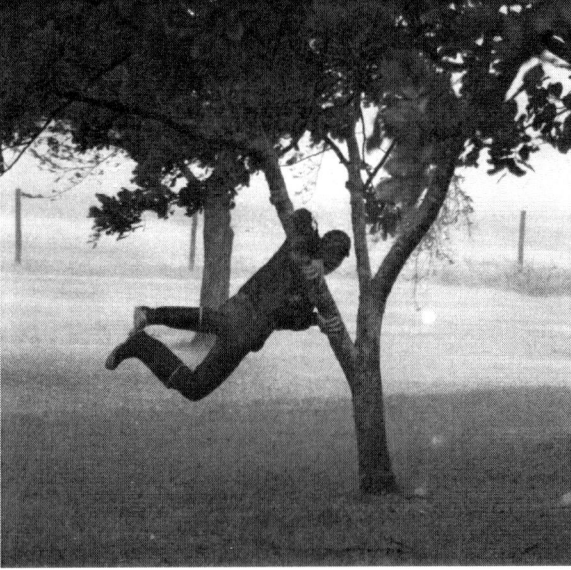

*Patient Connie's son, Ron, demonstrates how the Titus Family
survives all storms. And we agree with Thomas Paine who said,
"The harder the conflict, the more glorious the triumph."*

Courtesy of Photographer Neal Titus

Wednesday, January 12, 2005

Dear Doctor:

You, in your position, could probably write a book on how patients put their lives in order at the last minute. Read what I believe to be my last hoorah. I will skedaddle any time now.

The entire year of 2004 unfolded as my grand finale. I smile at every remembrance. I kid you not, each month presented itself chock-full of fervor, fun, and passion to the utmost factor. Tied-up loose ends, realized dreams, honored promises, recorded progress, and answered prayers are nifty ways to close a chapter.

January opened with a final decree on a long-time business concern, providing Neal with a bit of financial relief. I can't think of anyone who deserves it more. Maintaining my health has drained his wallet dry over the years. Our first two pleasures were replacing a leaky roof and constructing a screened porch off the family room. Unbeknownst to us, these two investments would shield us from roaring winds later in the year. We sometimes grumble over God's delays, but he always proves a method to his madness.

Our 1948 Chevrolet waited patiently for restoration since 1995. A wife's cancer squelches classic car enthusiasm. Motivation, strength, free time, money for car parts, and the fun of attending car shows took a dive. Hobby progress was hardly noticeable. But the beloved project came together in 2004. The engine cranked, original paint color coated the body, and authentic interior fashion took us back in time. Hand signals by a beaming gray-bearded driver wearing a fedora completed the '40s image, and we were off down the country road on a Sunday afternoon.

I hugged close three dear friends for the very last time.

Cancer took them up, up and away from my sight, causing my own plans for living to become more treasured.

Spots on my cheek were only basal cell, simulated heart attacks were simply esophageal spasms, and my sister's breast condition proved benign—all loud reasons to rejoice.

The Passion of the Christ [52] gripped a full theatre with dramatic silence. Truly, I think I sat through the entire film without breathing, yet my heartbeat raced. Sacrifice took on new implications, and souls revived with a united passionate desire to understand our one true God.

It is pleasing to see children work on personal and professional achievements. Our daughter and her husband bought their dream home where I had enough strength to strip wallpaper. Our son completed EMT training, the first phase of Firefighting Academy. His animation and love for clinical study kept us revved up each evening.

I turned half a century old. Men in white coats said I would never do it.

For sheer fun, my family and I stood nearby and feasted our eyes and ears on Bill Cosby—*live!*—and Earth, Wind & Fire—*live!* These gentlemen age beautifully and can still thrill large crowds. For two days in July I harmonized with a room full of professional vocalists at a Kempke Music Conference, a grand honor for this amateur, second-row alto. August 1 seemed like a good day to jump out of an airplane, so I did. And there you have five months full of elation.

Two fierce hurricanes tried to knock the livin' daylights out of our town, but we rolled with their punches and grew bigger, better, stronger. Townspeople now own a greater wisdom of what really matters.

Thanksgiving expressions were intense. Holy days humbled and modified themselves into something sweeter.

And my 2004 calendar was full to overflowing with dance. Reflection on this spectacular year leaves me wondering what could be better than this. But then maybe they've all been grand finales; I just failed to notice or claim God's kindness reserved for me.

"Once you were less than nothing; now you are God's own. Once you knew very little of God's kindness; now your very lives have been changed by it" (I Peter 2:10, TLB).

I've been changed by it, all right. Join me in a toast of champagne.

Connie

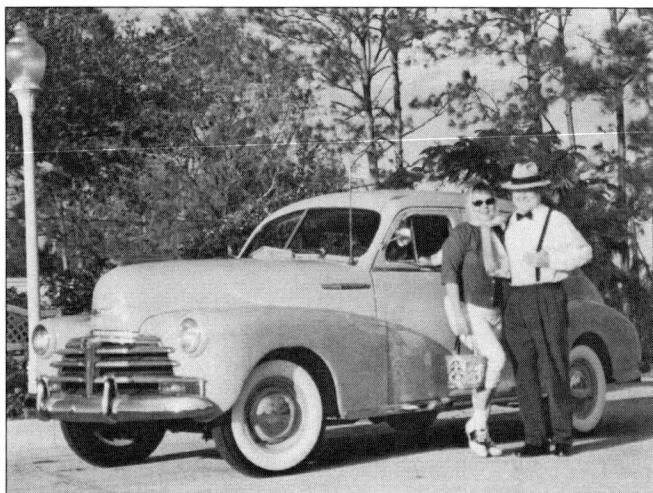

Patient Connie and Classic Lover-Man, Neal, stand beside their 1948 Chevrolet Stylemaster 4-door sedan named Babe.

Courtesy of Photographer Amy Milette

Wednesday, January 19, 2005

Good Day!

Or it would be, if you had not pissed me off yesterday. Honesty is good between us, right?

The whole idea of an office visit is for the patient to inform the doctor of concerns. Is this true or false? Proficient as I am, I presented myself yesterday with a typed page of body malfunction. As usual, you snatched the paper out of my hand, skimmed through at break-neck speed, and answered nothing. (And you wonder why I write some notes in code?)

What I got was a lecture. You seem to have an image of me pacing the house all day long, wringing my hands, fretting where and how soon the disease might strike again. And that I have nothing else to do. The word *panic* was part of your terminology in a horrid soapbox sermon. Talk about jumping to conclusions.

I beg your pardon, sir. Please see below how my body parts operate without panic. This takes five minutes to read. Have at it.

There is no time in my life for pacing, fretting, or panic. My feet hit the floor, I apply Revlon's Vintage Wine lipstick, and I go out into the world most every day of the week. I reach out and touch someone, anyone, with a word of love and grace. Patients ask me to escort them to doctors' appointments or treatments because I know how to laugh and walk on the lighter side. I cook meals for those who are sick or immobilized by surgery and sing to them whether I am in good voice or not.

I joined a Monday morning card ministry at our church where we write greetings to visitors, birthday and anniversary people, and those with prayer requests and/or joys. I conduct my own card and letter ministry, as you well know.

I take an active part in my children's lives, in all they say and do. When Mr. Titus pulls into the driveway at day's end, I am ready…wearing June Cleaver pearls and an apron. The Temptations sing "Night and Day."[53] We grab each other for a romantic dance. Neal whispers in my ear, "What did you do today, little girl?" I show him the pile of landscape timbers I dug up and sawed in half with the power saw. He then makes his way through the kitchen, nibbling on his Atkins veggie platter, peeking into the pot on the stove to see what's cookin'.

Now there are a few days nothing gets done, but more often than not, I push myself.

If I didn't panic stepping out of an airplane, how or why should I panic over symptoms in my body? I have taken everything in stride, held my head high with determination, and I am not afraid to die. Read my lips man-doctor. *I am not afraid to die!*

I do get sick and tired of two years' worth of drive-by shootings, as you call them, along with a host of other persistent head, neck, and chest glitches. And I lose patience over the fact that no physician within a thirty-mile radius has any inkling as to the reason or cause. Lord knows I can do without yesterday's implications, your chuckles, shaking head, shrugs, rolling eyes, or whispers to the nurses that I am loony, looking for trouble, or hungry for attention.

Panic does enter into the picture, however, if I see you fading from my corner of the ring, like yesterday. God, I hate that feeling.

Nevertheless, there is a plus side to your false images and the friction between us. When I am convinced you are not on the same page, nor do you know which book we are working from, I cry, which is cleansing. When you topple off that pedestal, shattering a jewel in your crown and proceed to stagger like a real person, I realize I must rely fully on God. Leadership titles shift. (I own a set of false images of you too, confusing you with someone you can never be.) Once I recognize the truth, my face turns to the Chief Physician and he saves me from your ruckus. "It is better to trust the Lord than to put confidence in men" (Psalm 118:8, TLB). Alan S. Collin's divinity strips away, leaving you a God-given, on-the-ground, tandem partner.

Additional goodness for us both: your human activity kindles more and more love in my heart. And it must be a relief of sorts when divine burden is removed from your shoulders. How about this? I'll practice patience until all the pieces of the *drive-by-shootings* puzzle fall into place. And they will. And you shall promise me no more panic sermons. Is it a deal?

I pray you will stay attached to me as any good tandem instructor. One day we will marvel at the finished puzzle, together.

Until then, love from your panic-less, skydiving IBC survivor,

Connie

P.S. While we talk on the subject of false images, currently there are commercials and newscasts that make me laugh out loud but also irritate me to no end. Procrit and Neulasta commercials are an insult to cancer patients' intelligence. Procrit commercials suggest you should call your doctor if you are on chemotherapy and feel tired. *Duh!* Neulasta commercials show a gentleman—a smiling, happy gentleman—running along the beach beside his dog, indicating his Neulasta shot made this possible. *Hogwash!* Producers omit the part of extreme bone pain. And what is all this hype about Herceptin being the new wonder drug? I tested for Herceptin in 1997. Herceptin is not new.

Thanks for letting me voice hogwash. Now all we have to do is inform the broadcasting system.

Wednesday, February 9, 2005

Dear Friend or Complete Stranger:

Yesterday I approached you with a topic we've danced around for years. Who knows why this subject matter comes spilling out of me now. Perhaps I face another crossroad and my best defense is reflecting on deep matters.

I asked about *your* relationship with God. One more time you soft-shoe tap-danced around the room trying to change the subject. But I changed it right back. You reasoned, "What matters here, Connie, what measures up in a patient's success, is *their* belief or faith, not mine." I stood in front of the doorknob, refusing to leave the cubicle without your honest response. You spoke your mind all right. "I believe in a higher, rather distant being or power, who has some degree of control and some influence in the world today." Period. My little inquisition ended abruptly. *Distant* and *some* are the two words that caused me to crumble.

I can just imagine the stunned, colorless look on my face. It would be easier to hear bad news about the cancer. Was my jaw dropped, brow furrowed? I know my eyes were wide and full of tears.

Oh, dear God! Dr. Collin! You caught me totally off guard, and in no way, at that deep-impact moment, could I verbally express my viewpoint, debate with you, or show you a better way. You obviously have gone astray. I could not get away from you fast enough. I sailed right past the checkout window, retreated with haste to my car, and cried my eyeballs out for the next twelve hours. No kidding. Who *are* you? Where is the spiritual hero I created you to be? After all this time and trial together, after working closely to accomplish hard work and speaking of each other with familiarity—for eight years—how could you revert back to a complete stranger in less than two minutes? I am not sure we can continue and be effective, or in tune.

In September 2002, I joined with a church group to read the Holy Bible from cover to cover. It was my first time. To shed light on God's Chosen People and to bring me closer to three Jewish friends (you and two delightful ladies), I chose and read a companion book, *What is a Jew?* by Rabbi Morris N. Kertzer, revised by Rabbi Lawrence A. Hoffman. Each chapter described you to a tee. I read your heart's business in this book, or so I thought.

Odd timing, don't you think? September 2002, was the beginning of those shooting pains in my head, the tingling and sore scalp. Reading God's Holy Word can be mind-boggling. But I think the head pain was a signal from God for me to stop confusing my Alan S. Collin with the men in the book, *What is a Jew?*

Do you want to know who I thought you were prior to yesterday (both you the man and you the doctor)? Below are quotes, highlights, and paraphrased clippings from Rabbi Kertzer's book that create an image of a man-doctor I truly love. And yes, I've been up all night typing.

• • •

My Alan S. Collin, M.D.

Jewish folklore revolves around my Alan S. Collin, M.D. He greets everyone cheerfully, gives them the benefit of the doubt, looks not at the bottle but at what it contains, and always begins a lesson with a humorous illustration. His traditional Jewish humor creates a wealth of laughter up and down the hallways.

In the words of Micah, my Alan S. Collin does justice, loves goodness, and walks humbly with his God. He gives generously to charities, supports organizations that work for peace, and votes for social programs that eliminate suffering and disease. Day-to-day, hour-by-hour, he practices deeds that are pleasing in the sight of God.

He acknowledges God as a real presence in the lives of

men and women, children and adults. He knows that reality as surely as he knows the beauty of love, the satisfaction of faithfulness, or the buoyancy of hope.

What my Alan S. Collin, M.D., believes about the Bible, about miracles, about a life after death is secondary to what he believes about the support he receives from God as he pursues his human potential and his basic moral responsibilities toward humanity. He knows all he is and all he has comes from God.

He accepts spiritual leadership in his family.

He is positive, not negative; he is open, not closed. My Alan S. Collin's life is a mixture of the ordinary and the profound, reminding him his existence can be beautiful or painful, but above all, inexplicable.

He believes that God created us with a physical and emotional need for each other, and he concurs with the Rabbis that sex is not only necessary, but desirable.

My Alan S. Collin's Jewish calendar encourages him to live to the fullest. He pauses to rejoice, to grieve, to apologize, and to celebrate. Some days are intensely personal, others communal, but all invite him to affirm his ties to family, friends, the Jewish people, and the world entire. He participates fully in all holidays and festivals.

Purim is a wild and public display of unrestricted joy, highlighted by carnivals and nonsense. Purim is a really good description of what goes on in Alan S. Collin's cancer clinic, all through the calendar year.

High Holy Days prompt him to return to God. He believes in the grand promise of atonement and forgiveness. My Alan S. Collin, M.D., sins, but he also knows moments when he does precisely what God wants, and does it well— even beyond his wildest imagination. Reconciliation is achieved by an honest searching of his soul, a candid admission of his shortcomings, and a firm resolution to bridge the gap between what he is and what he knows he should be.

Chanukah celebrates the light of home, rededication, and God's miraculous presence in his life.

Every relationship, every ambition means more to my Alan S. Collin if it is clothed in some symbolic act. Rituals lend poetry to life; they provide inner passion—from the food he eats to the very passing of time. He believes human nature is in flux; people grow constantly in life, and as they do, rituals are likely to change.

My Alan S. Collin's ideal meal is shared with friends and family. It is an opportunity dedicated to deepening relationships and expressing thanks to God. He believes in the guidance, solace, and wisdom of Torah; therefore, words of Torah pass across his table often. God's spirit then dwells in his home.

Sabbath (Shabbat) is a time for my Alan S. Collin, M.D., to refresh spiritually. As his family sits down on Sabbath, candles are lit, special songs are sung, and prayers are offered. He praises God for the week past, for life and strength, for home and love and friendship, for the discipline of trials and temptations, for the happiness that has come to him out of his labors. He feels God ennobles him with work and love. He trusts his life is not in vain and that he makes a difference in the lives of others.

He uses the occasion of the Sabbath to invoke God's blessings on his children. His children grow from childhood to adulthood, and because the years pass by so quickly, each stage of their journey is important to him.

A wedding is always sheer delight for my Alan S. Collin, M.D. He shines in an active role. In fact, I understand that back in his longhaired days, he attended a wedding celebration and somehow ended up dancing around topless. Sounds like Purim's wild and public display of unrestricted nonsense again, or is it one of the seven wedding blessings that a longhaired Jewish hematologist/oncologist do a wild, unrestricted topless dance? At any rate, everyone in the office has a snapshot of his antics pasted on their refrigerator. I wait patiently for my copy.

His best advice to the bride and groom is that they should rejoice together and sacrifice for each other willingly, sharing life's burdens as they are encountered.

Even though my Alan S. Collin, M. D., builds his financial empire, he agrees with Jewish tradition emphasizing simplicity—especially at weddings and funerals—because all people are equal in God's sight. There should be no distinction on the basis of creed, color, gender, or class. He believes all men and women are together a single family with a single destiny.

His oncology work is immersed in life and death on a daily basis. Below is my Alan S. Collin's sound doctrine on life and death.

Because of his innate trust in God, he affirms the value of life and life's pleasures. Human life is sacred and filled with the promise of the ultimate reign of God. Life is good, precious, and holy, yet my Alan S. Collin, M.D., understands the suffering folks go through and feels a dignified death is also a good and precious thing.

He strengthens the bond of people-hood through his vocation. He wants to be his brother's or sister's keeper.

My Alan S. Collin, M.D., nudges each patient into a union with God. He teaches that God is as close as our breathing. Pain and anxiety can be replaced by the surety and radiance of God's close and abiding love.

He agrees that death is fully determined by the Lord our God, not Alan S. Collin, M.D. When death of a family member or patient friend is inevitable, he finds consolation in the Kaddish prayer. This prayer makes it easier to let go of life with all its treasures because these things are not and never have been ours. When a sunset, a bird's song, a baby's smile, the thunder of music, surge of great poetry, or a heart's dream slips from our hands, we can well trust them to the hands of God who made them.

My Alan S. Collin honors the dead. Those who were once alive should never be forgotten or treated with disrespect.

My Alan S. Collin, M.D., was taught that God is to be worshipped out of love. He respects the honest, devout worshipper of any faith. There are many paths to one God. Likewise there are many direct and simple ways to worship—not just in fancy synagogues but in the woods or while walking along a country lane. My Alan S. Collin regards three places sacred—his synagogue, his home, and the land of Israel. Much of his worship takes place around his table with family and friends.

He praises God for creation, revelation, and redemption. He prays for wisdom, for health, and peace. My Alan S. Collin, M.D., prays for a day when all humanity shall come to serve God. His prayers may not be fancy, but they are shaped by a devout spirit.

My Alan S. Collin believes in redemption for the world, and he works to instill in every single human being the best that God has given them. His world rests on three foundations: justice, truth, and peace. He says if we deal justly with other people, truth will triumph and peace will reign. His most important ideals are thanksgiving, freedom, learning, sacrifice, and repentance. Freedom is to be prized above all.

The State of Israel is not only the Jewish ancestral home, but the birthplace of my Alan S. Collin's faith and his Bible. He supports the State of Israel financially and spiritually. He makes religious pilgrimages to see the miracle homeland, but as an American Jew, his political loyalty is to the United States.

Judaism and Christianity is a union that can break and rejoin and intertwine. My Alan S. Collin, M.D., honors his heritage and feels compassion for centuries of its suffering, persecution, and emotional barriers. And for a while his family preferred not to venture into the Gentile world, even if the gates were open. But he and his people unlearn quickly. He promotes Jews and Christians developing a partnership based on mutual respect and profound understanding. God will surely bless us all.[54]

• • •

This concludes the man I created you to be, the man-doctor I love. But who are you now, after yesterday's confession? Could you please take out your green Magic Marker and draw an arrow next to statements that apply? Are there any besides the one regarding sex?

I should probably look beyond book images and seek genuine character when choosing spiritual heroes. I would not want you forming any opinions about me and my character from a Methodist publication *The Book of Worship for Church and Home.* [55]

In Ruth Rosen's book *Jewish Doctors Meet the Great Physician*, a paragraph written by Dr. Jack J. Sternberg, medical oncologist in Little Rock, Arkansas, reminded me of me. Dr. Sternberg told of a woman patient with terminal breast cancer. This woman knew she would soon leave her husband widowed and her children motherless, but she seemed more concerned about her doctor's separation from God. The doctor couldn't get over the fact that God allowed disease to ravage this lady's body, yet she still loved, worshipped, and followed him. The licensed professional was overwhelmed.[56]

Is my licensed professional overwhelmed? I pray so.

Shalom from a Gentile friend,

Connie

Connie

Dear Friend:

In my last letter you were a complete stranger. May I address you as friend again?

Our conversation of last week haunts me still. I weep and shudder. And because it is on my mind twenty-six hours a day, I could not escape a vivid nighttime dream. No Cajun-style bean soup was involved this time. I did increase the intake of Darvocet for discomfort in my neck and chest. Does Darvocet invite active dreaming?

Last night I dreamed about you all night. Potty breaks did not interrupt this dramatic play. I awakened remembering clear details and replayed every bit of it for Neal. Nothing shocks him anymore. You've heard my crazy dreams, too. Do you want to hear this one?

You were my guest at a lavish banquet. I ushered you over to the endless, catered table, guiding you through the line. You started dishing yourself small meager amounts. I corrected you by taking your hand and dipping the serving spoon deep into the bowls for big, healthy portions. I, however, took limited helpings for myself because I knew many hungry people followed. We found our way to a table to partake of the feast and spirited fellowship.

After the meal, I led you upstairs to a large upper room. You and I and all the people in this upper room were wearing raincoats. What is the significance of raincoats? God only knows. The people in this upper room were my loving family of faith, those still living and those dearly departed. You sat in your raincoat on a sideline bench, watching and drinking in all the sounds and action of God's interactive love. I kept one eye on you and your enjoyment. End of dream.

One of my favorite hymns is, "Here I Am, Lord." Each time I sing it, I remember this dream and my faucet proceeds to leak. People in my pew inquire about my tears, but they would never understand, so I ask them for a tissue. Excerpts of this tear-jerking lyrical story follow:

> The Lord of sea and sky has heard his people cry. The Lord of snow and rain has borne his people's pain. Finest bread he will provide, 'til their hearts be satisfied, he will set a feast for them—whom shall he send? Refrain: Here I am, Lord. Is it I, Lord? I have heard you calling in the night. I will go, Lord, if you lead me, I will hold your people in my heart.[57]

I have heard God calling in the night with a feast and raincoat dream. I think of you and continually wonder what my elongated life is supposed to accomplish. Am I to invite you to a feast set by God, dish you up food for thought in large portions, shield you with a raincoat, invite you to an upper room, wash your feet, or dance you around in a crowd of noisy but very loving Methodists?

Perhaps.

I know one thing for sure—if I had this dream prior to our conversation on February 8, it would mean nothing. No Kleenex necessary. But it does mean something. I offer my extended hand. Be my guest. I will pick you up at 7:00 p.m.

Love,

Connie

Connie, your banquet hostess

Tuesday, February 22, 2005

Dr. Collin:

Apparently I am good at cancer. Here we go again. Another recurrence. Number five. As I shimmy over your threshold, Neil Diamond sings "Hello Again."[58] Olivia Newton John adds that maybe I hang around here a little more than I should.[59]

My total body massage on January 27 soothed and relaxed me as usual. But the next day, the mysterious shooting pains in my head stepped up in voltage, localizing behind my right ear. This is no exaggeration. I experienced ten to fifteen sharp pains each and every minute and felt no other choice but to climb into bed with Darvocet. My sister insisted I call you immediately; my rule of thumb is that if I still suffer in seven days, I will go see about it. Turns out, Day Seven was my worst day, so I broke down and made two phone calls—one to you and your scan scheduling staff and one to a neurologist who hopefully could get to the bottom of unexplained head pain.

MRIs of the head and cervical spine and a PET scan were scheduled. I saw a neurologist and he suggested my head pains, tingling, and sore scalp are normal responses to radiation and chemo treatments gone by. He can easily put me on seizure medication to settle them down. Gee. Doctors love to load patients up with medicine.

Drive-by-shootings become another signal. Join me for a short vignette.

Did you see the movie *Apollo 13*[60] with Tom Hanks? Picture the control room of NASA placed in heaven. Ed Harris' character is God. God (Ed Harris) orders one of his technicians wearing horned-rimmed glasses and a starched, short-sleeved white shirt to sit down at the control booth and zap Mrs. Connie Titus on Windemere Drive with ten volts behind the right ear until she calls her oncologist. Each day God (Ed Harris) checks with the control technician. "Anything yet? Did she call the doctor? How is she responding—what is she saying?"

The horned-rimmed, goofy-looking genius reports, "She is on a steady diet of Darvocet and bed rest, and she told her sister she would see about it in seven days. Darvocet every eight hours is not holding her pain."

On Thursday, February 7, God (Ed Harris) becomes impatient and shouts to increase the voltage to fifteen. At 3:00 p.m. the technician is happy to report that Mrs. Connie Titus on Windemere Drive followed through with God's plan. Phone calls were made. Appointments were in place. God smiled and ordered the machine to be shut down. And the intense pain behind the right ear vanished, disappeared.

I usually steer clear of patterns, but this time a pattern unfolded. Just like two years ago, you called on a Friday to tell me the MRI of the brain was clear. Just like two years ago, you called on the following Wednesday to report the PET scan revealed a problem. Just like two years ago, you ordered more testing.

Hopeful key words on current reports are *early, small, and new* because we caught it with God's voltage. The plan is to begin chemotherapy, the same two drugs that worked two years ago. But first I need another infusaport planted into my chest. Oh, joy.

I am relieved in three ways. (What other patient says she's relieved her cancer has recurred?) 1. I don't have to say I feel good when I do not. 2. No longer will I go, go, go, or answer yes, yes, yes to multiple committees. 3. I feel in tune with the Maker of my body. He and I communicate effectively. That is the best part.

Regarding Item #2, a cancer patient claims the right to go, go, go with activities of her choice. My red-plaid friend visited weekend before last. Tree houses are significant to our younger days and, wouldn't you know it, Mr. Titus and I own one. At least I think it is still a tree house. During last year's hurricanes my husband and son stored crap beneath this structure: wood planks and logs, full five-gallon buckets of paint, an old muffler, a huge metal tailgate, a few empty beer bottles, and a snake, to boot. Before my friend's visit I single-handedly removed all this crap; prepped and painted the wood inside and out; and added potted flowers, a wind chime and homemade cushions. My red-plaid friend and I climbed up onto our cushions, drank White Russians made with ice cream, ate strawberries dipped in chocolate, and told many secrets. This is pretty darn good for a dame tainted with cancer.

I will meet with you, sir, after my port is in place. Please stay healthy, happy, and safe until then. You must be fit in order to fix me.

It is good to need you so.

Connie

Connie

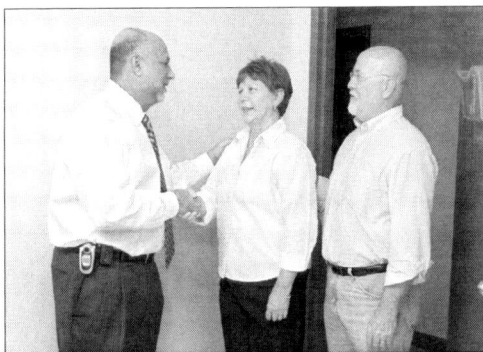

Patient Connie and Husband Neal greet once more a medicine man by the name of Dr. Collin. They must map out a strategic plan for curtailing Patient's fifth recurrence.

Courtesy of Photographer Jerry Brewer

Friday, March 4, 2005

Happy Birthday, Alan S. Collin, M.D.:

You might not appreciate this birthday card. It's a Kodak moment of an old, yet virile and enthusiastic gentleman, probably in his late 70s. He dons only a pair of swimming trunks and his prescription eyeglasses. He proceeds to show off for two elderly, heavy-set women dressed in their extra-large purple and pink bathing suits. They sit on the beach in front of him, dazzled by his performance. He completes numerous deep knee bends, holding his arms out straight, focusing on the horizon. His audience of two applauds and smiles. They've never seen anything quite like it before.

"Nothing great was ever achieved without enthusiasm!"[61]

That's my sister Judy in purple. She always sits on my right at the beach. And I'm in pink, size 2X. See our appreciation? Bravo. Bravo. We are feasting our eyes on those pecs, the flexibility in your knees, your balance, and focus. Wowee!

Remember when you and I talked the other day about you being the best man you've ever been right now? Well, here you are.

My sister and I must also applaud your Maker, your Counselor and Sustainer. The biblical text of 1 Chronicles, chapter 29 states that God alone brings you to this season of excellence and we believe this to be true. He fashions you into an agile dazzler. He stokes your charms to delight folks of any age, stage, gender, or hair color. Thanks for following along with his plan for you and for us. Your season of excellence is equivalent to a bright light, and that light keeps your patients warm on the way to their miracles.

...O Lord...We adore you as being in control of everything. Riches and honor come from you alone, and you are the Ruler of all mankind; your hand controls power and might, and it is at your discretion that men are made great and given strength

1 Chronicles 29:11b-12 (TLB)

Your fifty-fifth birthday is a grand time to compliment one's dazzle effect. How did we do?

Love from,

Connie

Connie in pink, Judy in purple

P.S. We are glad your back and knees are strong to hoist us sturdy old ladies up off our bums.

But first, wait, what can you offer as an encore? Do you dance at this age? I bet so.

Tuesday, March 22, 2005

Commander in Chief:

Whenever you and I concur on a plan, survivorship strengthens. With this new batch of cancer, we agreed a little more Navelbine and a little more Xeloda should do the trick as they did in 2003. Let us begin again.

I came alone this morning—no big deal. I am a professional now. You took my hand and led me to the chemo room. I asked you to seat me in either Jane or Dorothy's favorite chair. The blank look on your face sent my emotions reeling.

You asked, "Who?" Now, that was a big, sad deal.

"Oh, no, oh no! Dr. Collin! What is the matter with you? You know who, Jane and Dorothy—two of your beloved patients, two of your best cheerleaders and character references, two important miracle ladies who made my treatments in 2003 an absolute hootenanny. They both died within the year. Come on, guy. Don't tell me you have forgotten them already. Is this how you are?"

If one of my current Tuesday morning chemo buddies has a recurrence within a year of my death and asks to be seated in Connie's favorite chair, will you stare blankly into space and mutter, "Connie? Connie who?"

Tell me it isn't so. My head swims with the idea that patients possibly mean nothing to you.

I sat down in Dorothy's favorite chair, next to Jane's favorite chair, and tried out Dr. Cappelletti's brand new infusaport. The good news is we got an immediate blood return. I cried buckets over your flippant detachment, but at the same time I replayed lively conversations of my two fancy friends.

We were the three musketeers together, don't you remember? You were at your best with Jane and Dorothy. They passed the baton to me to jazz up this chemo suite. I missed them in the worst way today. Now I miss you. Who are you?

Where have you hidden my caring physician who commemorates dearly departed patients?

I failed Jane and Dorothy with hot tears and muffled curse words. No three-ring circus today.

But wait. (Drum roll, please.) Nurse Cathy saved the day in Wonder Woman fashion. The circus came to town after all.

An old gentleman and his wife sat across from me in the chemo room. I think his name is Walter. Nurses favored Walt. His face was pale, very pale. Come to find out, his lower blood pressure number only registered forty. With careful monitoring, you all were trying to decide whether or not to send him to the hospital by way of squad. Once more Nurse Cathy caught you in the hallway, reporting on this sweet man. She carried a loaded shot in her hand. Chemo patrons overheard Nurse Cathy confidently and playfully command you to, "Bend over!"

And of course your reply was, "In your dreams!"

Well, you should have heard us natives chanting over Cathy's suggestion. I have to say, we were on board. Grand idea, Cathy!

Thirty minutes later, you made an appearance in the chemo room, checking on certain patients, especially Walt with weak pressure. He rested comfortably, outstretched in his recliner with a warm blankie.

It was my turn. Nurse Nicole and Nurse Cathy worked with me. You joined us. Bent over, you listened to my heart and lungs and then plastered the stethoscope to my forehead, hoping to hear secret thoughts, I suppose. Cathy's whimsical plan came up again, in my thoughts and out loud. "Yeah, bend over."

All chaired participants, a group undivided, began this savage jeering that elevated in volume. With a serious expression I have never before seen on your face, you quickly straightened up and backed away out of our intentions (beep, beep, beep), until you just about tripped over Walt's footrest and sat down in his lap. That would be one way to raise his blood pressure.

You are one comical circus act, buddy. Oh, the benefits of belly laughter. White cells elevated around our savage circle.

Yes, in our survivor dreams we would love to: inject, into our oncologist, a high dose of his strongest chemo cocktail (arm wrestling to see who gets the honor); cut essential, beloved body parts from, or insert foreign objects into our surgeon; scope the gastroenterologist; dig out a basal cell from the face of a handsome plastic surgeon; and reach in with rubber gloves and pluck something deep in the belly of a male gynecologist, while smiling.

This might be a good place to inform you of something. Are you aware that most of your chemo nurses are deathly afraid of needles? What the heck is wrong with this picture?

Anyway, our most pleasing privilege would be scheduling scans and nuclear tests for physicians (and nurses) every three months, so you all can collect and enjoy (by way of needles) a wide array of contrast chemical materials, the kind that make us glow in the dark and isolate us from babies and/or pregnant women. Did you see William Hurt in *The Doctor*?[62] Just like that.

Bend over, sir. Make our dreams come true.

You know? I am in quite a predicament here. Essential for my good health and well-being is seeing you on a frequent, regular basis. But in order to see you, pick up revised dance steps, or nestle in your strong arms on a frequent, regular basis, I must be sick with disease.

There has to be a solution. Surrender. Is surrender the solution? I cannot put my finger on it right now, but I think it was my friend J. Ellsworth Kalas who said: "Genuine surrender says, 'Father, if this problem, pain, sickness is needed to fulfill your purpose and glory in my life or in another's, please don't take it away!'" Ooh, I must be careful what I pray for, right? But please, Father, don't take my thorn away because

I no longer would require the playful company of Alan S. Collin, M.D., P.A.

Signed,

Connie

Connie Beth Thompson Titus

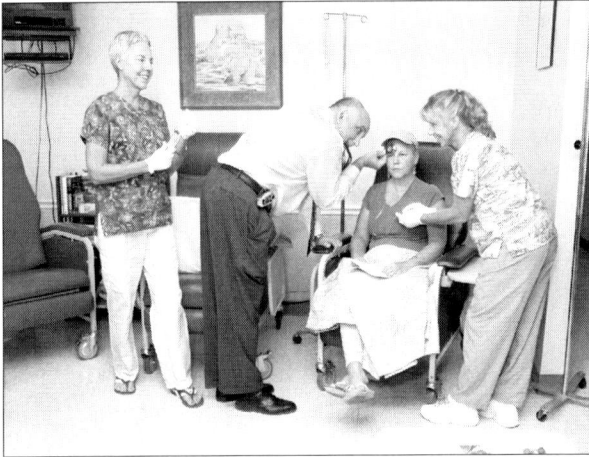

Dr. Collin reads Patient Connie's thoughts with his stethoscope while Nurse Nicole and Nurse Cathy conspire on how to give the good Doctor a taste of his own medicine.

Courtesy of Photographer Jerry Brewer

• • •

Tale by the Sea

By the seaside God calls me by name. My given name is plain ol' Connie Beth, not Constance Elizabeth. Boy, am I glad. Constance Elizabeth brings to mind a self-sufficient woman who might not need a Savior the way Connie Beth does. "…I have called you by name; you are mine" (Isaiah 43:1, TLB).

Friday, September 9, 2005

Dear Dr. Collin,

Neal and I are sorry to hear of your father's passing. I keep thinking of you walking around with a hole in your heart while the world spins and folks depend upon you. My mom and dad died over twenty years ago, so I know firsthand what it's like. Perhaps one day soon you and I could have a few quiet moments. Talk to me about your father—about his character, his interests and occupation, what was important to him, and the inner workings of your father/son relationship. Please know I care. I want to carry a floodlight into your hurting world.

Love from a light bearer,

Connie

• • •

Two Tales by the Sea

Last week I photographed a favored combination: sunrise, the beach, and my Bible entitled *The Way*. My photograph came back from the developer with a rather interesting touch. A large sphere of light hung over the book. Professional photographers or developers cannot give me a practical reason for this strange ball of mist or whatever. The cover on my Bible is not shiny so it is not a reflection. There was no mist in the air, no raindrops on the lens. I took the negative in for thirty reprints, thinking they'd make unique greeting cards. But the developer darkened them, trying to fix the problem. I returned them, telling the developer I like the problem ball of light and asked him to please put the problem back the way it was. That day I read about the Creator of light and his intentions. "…the mercy of our God is very tender, and heaven's dawn is about to break upon us, to give light to those who sit in darkness and death's shadow, and to guide us to the path of peace" (Luke 1:78-79, TLB).

On another occasion, Mr. Titus arose early to photograph me dancing at the beach. I instructed him how to use my Olympus Stylus 120/35 mm camera, which produced run-of-the-mill, uneventful early dawn portraits. But he also took a few shots with his new toy—a digital camera. Each digital clip showed a small orange ball of light on me or near me. Neal apologized for the flaw. Could the unexplained sphere of light over *The Way* be related to Neal's small orange ball of light on me or near me?

Symbolic possibilities leave me speechless, although you'd not know it with the size of this tale! There is no flaw, reflection, or mistake in photo development. As I walk or dance, stand or swim, or study at my peak place for growth, God's grace and character form into an unexplained sphere or ball of light. His spirit illumines me, fills dark corners, and guides me to a path of peace. "If you are filled with light within, with no dark corners, then your face will be radiant too, as though a floodlight is beamed upon you" (Luke 11:36, TLB).

Tuesday, October 4, 2005

Dr. Collin, Sir:

Tall, dark, handsome Physician Assistant Steve Riley follows your every move. Why? What are you up to? You are not getting ready to retire, are you? Remember, patients with several four-inch charts must approve all personnel changes.

Regarding my lower abdomen pain since mid-July, you speculated aloud whether or not I encountered a bedpost or doorjamb. Are we talking about a bump and grind type of thing? You are excellent proof that a man thinks about sex every six minutes, or is it six seconds? Anyway, after the colonoscopy, pelvic ultrasound, bone scan, pelvic X-ray, CA-125, and PAP smear all proved cancer free, I searched my archives for possible bedpost or doorjamb injuries.

Okay, yes. Twenty-nine years ago this week I encountered a doorjamb. Early Friday morning, October 1, 1976, I refused to let Neal transport me to the hospital until our neighbor across the street, Gwen Robinson, went to work. She would see us leaving with packed Lamaze bag, assume it was another false alarm, and call the whole neighborhood. I waited, waited for her to go to work until I literally climbed the front doorjamb with desperate labor pain. I didn't know Gwen Robinson had the day off. We made it to the hospital somehow; our daughter was born two hours later.

Bedposts? I sold Neal's four-poster waterbed out from underneath him last fall. We slept in that bed for probably twenty years. I don't ever remember my abdomen coming in contact with a bedpost, by accident or on purpose. Jamie Lee Curtis in *True Lies* [63] I am not. Sorry.

So my lower abdomen discomfort continues and will remain a mystery, I suppose, like shooting head pains, tingling, and sore scalp going on three years now. It is just part of the wonderfulness of me. Put Steve Riley to work on it. He is probably still concerned about your bedpost and doorjamb theory.

Have you got any other IBCers with abdomen pain I can compare myself to?

Connie

Friday, October 21, 2005

Dr. Collin:

In between office visits I write letters, which you fling like Frisbees toward the citrus box and then Nurse Alice has to come in and clean up behind you. You got me started on dancing and musical dreaming and such. Are you ready for this one? Listen first to what my friend Joni says.

> I experience this bittersweet sadness with intimate friends. I love them so much that I want to pass through them, reach the other side, know them fully. Not to possess them but to meld with them. I can't on earth. I'm on the outside of their heart's door, always wanting to get in, get closer, even while relishing their company. My longings are eased knowing that in heaven, I will "get in."[64]

Dr. Collin, what is it about you that entices me to *get in?*

• • •

Countless hours we sit alone together in a cubicle, our room of practice. You and I, a duet, look over the score. Daytime serenade begins. Will there be harmony or offbeat discord today? Too often we behave like out-of-tune strangers.

Movement One: Discord

You waltz in imitating a physician. I must look like a chart number or dollar sign to you—dressed in a blue paper sack. That starched white coat you wear places you up on a level I can never, ever reach...not even on tiptoe.

Each office visit begins with the same unspoken prelude, a ballad burning in my heart.

Me: "How do I get in? How will I know?"

You: "Get in where? How will you know what, darlin'?"

Me: "How do I get in closer? How will I know if you are sick or sad or lonely? How will I know if you've gone astray and I am someone to show the way?"

You: "It is not the job of a second row alto to worry over the bandmaster."

Oh. No rumba again today. You prescribe dancing, but not with you, I guess.

Flipping through my overgrown chart, you rattle off questions with your back turned toward me, exercising your lyrical authority. I cannot seem to form one intelligent response. Then I ask the questions. Your solutions are not at all what I expect to hear; therefore, I forget them immediately.

Turning to face me, finally, you put on your vaudeville hat. And I laugh. Not that I understand your slapstick humor, but because you are a delightful spectacle in motion.

It's time to lie back on the cold, hard table. My blue paper crackles. I strain hard to hear at least some elevator music. You touch me in all the familiar places—a rhythmic, yet sterile, mindless exam. And I am numb. So tell me again, how does mindless and numb combine to identify any new problem?

You wash me down the drain with anti-bacterial soap while I flounder to sit up. I am flat on one side, crackled, and now jumbled. A few comments are scratched onto a 3-ply form. I sense you and your vaudeville act are about to exit.

"Hey, you, wait a minute. Come closer," I initiate today's embrace. It is an awkward, stiff sort of movement. Two off-beat, out-of-tune strangers bounce off each other.

That's all, folks. Jam session is over for another three months. The door opens. You disappear into dead silence, Stage Right.

God, I needed more.

Movement Two: Mystery

My medical history is a mystery from start to finish, yes? Here is more proof. Mysteriously, the split second I step across the threshold and walk away from you in the opposite direction, you enter me completely. A symphonic intercourse takes place, right there in the hallway on Nottingham Avenue.

Picture a scene from a special effects film. Listen for a

resonance, the dramatic musical crescendo of "Adagio for Strings"—none other will do. A brilliant, bright-colored, pulsating ball of vapor rushes for flat and jumbled me, Stage Left. *Shhhwwwhhooooosh…zzzziipp.*

You are in there, inside of me, melding. Your body, your mind, soul, and spirit…your size ten brown loafers, argyle socks, sapphire ring, and crooked forefingers…those gray whiskers, the joke you just told, and your Billy Joel eyes…I get it all.

Patients #2, #3, and #4 peer out to see what the commotion is. Thirteen waiting room patients and their caregivers transform into the string section of "Adagio for Strings."[65] Nurses stand in the aftermath whirlwind at Stage Right, scratching their heads. "Where is the doctor? He was here, in good measure, a moment ago."

I turn with a wink. "He's with me. You'll have to find another conductor to orchestrate these waiting patients," and through the revolving door with a bolt we go. A smuggler, I am.

But you are not the stranger I just bounced against in the cubicle. You are my other gray-bearded friend and lover.

Final Overture: Harmony

I know everything there is to know about you—what you are going to say, before you say it, and how you will look saying it. Your back does not turn toward me. You face me… front and center…attentive, interested, and curious. Genuinely, I laugh at your jokes from the inside out. Questions and answers flow back and forth, with sensual clarity or not. But we're in tune with a simple glance. And the band plays on.

How does a second row alto profess to know everything there is to know about the bandmaster? From 9-5 on weekdays, I nestle in the breast pocket of your white coat—adopting the rhythm of your heartbeat and respiration as my own, participating in your interaction with people like me, becoming an integral part of your response to them, your stamina, and your love of the practice. I get in and keep your music playing.

What shall we do at dusk? Let there be more melding and music, please. You show me to a second-story screened porch. Two Adirondack chairs face each other, close, touching. We sit all propped up with each other, simultaneously massaging stocking feet, sipping true cocktails, and confiding, in that order.

There is no sex. Sorry. I never quite learned the art of making love, nor could I bear any one-breasted grimace on your face. Besides, that's not what we are about, you and me.

Music can be our sex. Our midnight music in the moonlight is endorsed by Dr. Seuss. Be prepared to cut a rug in slow motion and harmonize 'til the wee hours. Earth, Wind & Fire's "That's the Way of the World,"[66] James Ingram/ Patty Austin's "How Do You Keep the Music Playing?",[67] and Peobo Bryson's rendition of "Silent Night."[68]

What? Can a Jewish man slow dance to a Christmas lullaby in mid-summer—a lullaby for the one I believe to be our Messiah? Are you allowed?

Neighbors are tempted to call the authorities by now, especially when Abraham, Isaac, Jacob, Harriet Beecher Stowe, and John and Charles Wesley come on the scene. Judaism and Methodism blend on that second-story porch. It's a mixed bag of worship with timbrel, lyre, and bagpipe. Bring in more Adirondack chairs, distilled liquid, maybe Earth, Wind & Fire.

We host a forum. Our night is far from silent. You and I and the ancestors enter into a spiritual encounter. At last, a close informal talk about Jehovah. I've waited many moons.

Forum conclusion: The same God who watches over the House of Jacob watches over the Beecher Family and then some. Secret prayers strike a major chord between us. Expression is pure and music is moving in this melding business.

Dr. Kalas tells me that you, a Jew, are the Tree of God, the Tree of Life, and I, a Gentile, am a wild shoot grafted on.[69] No wonder you are worn out after our office visits... dragging a wild Gentile around. An image comes to mind of a small child standing on Daddy's shoes as he dances through daily life. And wouldn't you know, at this very imaginary moment, I catch a glimpse of our Messiah, seated among us in an Adirondack chair. He keeps time to the music. I've told you this before, my Hebrew friend. You make him seem so real to me.

The sun rises. Day breaks. One more dance? You and I are no longer out-of-tune strangers. Discord turns to harmony in three easy movements. Melding is the ticket. I usher you back to the clinic where people with missing body parts have put away their violins and wait patiently for the doctor. Let us prescribe for them, too, dancing at daybreak. I've grown quite fond of the idea.

Passing through, reaching the other side, getting in, grafting, even melding with music is possible here on earth. It works for me. I must tell Joni.

Please behave, Alan S. Collin, M.D. Don't forget, I am in your breast pocket.

From discord...through mystery... into harmony...with you,

Connie

Connie

Monday, November 7, 2005

Dear Piano-Playing Medicine Man,

"Looking back we've touched on sorrowful days…you will find peace of mind if you look way down in your heart and soul…."[70]

What keeps my music playing, prevents my song from fading too fast, and brings me peace of mind? I look way down into my heart and soul.

Back in 1997 you told me that survivors survive by individual means. Revitalization happens in diverse measure, and one must privately discover what keeps his or her music playing. Neal concurs by encouraging me to do whatever blows the wind up my skirt. Read the stanzas of my surviving life, my verses and lyrics. See what blows the wind up my skirt and keeps my music playing.

• • •

Intro

Belly laughs in Room #3; fine-tuning; grit, valor, vigor, and amusement; signs; red-plaid memories; gray-bearded nursemaids with Christ-like character; granted good sense; encores; a groove in my shoes; a pair of new eyes; cold beer and a buzz saw; settling down and daylight.

Moderately, with Spirit

Flashing (the playful kind); giving orders; drop-kicking; grilled cheese sandwiches by candlelight; 8.6 cm dreams; fall foliage dusted with freshly fallen snow; physicians changing light bulbs; whimsy; majestic thunderclouds; a long boardwalk; protection from aliens; genuine interaction and honesty.

Very Simply and Expressively

Fences with strawberries; agreement and hope, even if it is a misunderstanding; gyrating intros; fiddles or bassoons and brass; jingling charms; sparkling stars; islanders vs. cows; big brotherhood; interchangeable roles; washing of feet and communion.

Fast and Lively

Strong pressure drawn from big hot water tanks; fountains, streams, and rivers at eventide; deep-sea diving/mountain-climbing women friends; microchips and wildlife; high promises to an only son; an enchanting, vintage daughter in love with a favorite son-in-law; strong hands holding a beating heart; zucchini bread, poked and prodded.

Very Gently, But Not Dragging

The Lord of sea and sky, snow and rain, wind and flame; impossible possibilities; open gates; an easy chair, melody, and fine wine in the darkness; syncopation; wild shoots grafting on; argyle socks; confiding; motivation; dazzling posture and a nurse heading for the doctor's behind with a very long needle in hand.

Firmly

Mr. Tentmaker's sensitivities; a Holy Spirit who is willing to work in and through human-ness; "...the simple-minded made wise!" (Proverbs 1:4, TLB); the wise made simple-minded; people holding hands around a table; smuggling and nestling now and again; dancing in the moonlight with Ella and Frank.

Gaiety

Lists written in code; knowing everything there is to know about the Bandmaster; reprieves; vibrant beach umbrellas and chairs at the plateau; silence; tales and tails by the sea; dynamic imagery; life forms; sensual beach rocks; blushing surgeons; White Russians made with ice cream and secrets in tree houses.

Quietly, with Feeling

Bonding of people; a glimpse of the Messiah within reach; ladies in yellow survivor shirts; encouraging words first thing in the morning; blond and brunette sisters; a whistling Patch Adams; grand finales; planting flower seeds and growing pearls.

• • •

You, my good man, Alan S. Collin, M.D., helped me write these lyrics, you penciled in the dynamics and composed the tunes I dance to. More recitals are scheduled, so I press on, I practice and strive to be even better. "Not that I have already obtained all this, or have already been made perfect, but I press on…" (Philippians 3:12, NIV).

With love and thanksgiving,

Connie

Sunday, November 27, 2005

Oh, Mentor of Mine:

How do I get off this stage? There seems no end to my story. I hear the music and keep it playing, but must I dance forever?

A telephone rings in the comfort of our daughter's home—one hundred twenty-two miles away. I answer. The call is for me. It is you.

Our topic of conversation includes positive hyper-metabolic accumulation in cervical and mediastinal lymph node groups in a pattern typical of malignancy, metastatic disease, a new finding.

Despite ongoing metastatic mindset, my heart races as if hearing the news for the very first time.

Between scans and results…in preparation…with hindsight… a strong urge to raise the white flag controls me. I want to inform my family and my doctor I will do nothing this time, and see.

Oh, but the human body, the human mind and soul are so very frail.

A husband's continual affirmation knocks around in my soul. "Thank you for being here, it's important to me."

How can I not try…for him?

Chemo cocktails are served straight up at 2:15 p.m. on a Friday. It must be Happy Hour somewhere in the world. Strangers are present in your absence.

You are a canticle of light in my darkness, even when you're invisible.

This is not over until you sing with the fat lady.

And then, dear man, you may dance with me, Cliff Huxtable[71] style, right down off this stage.

Thank you and goodnight,

Connie

Connie

Tuesday, August 15, 2006

Dr. Collin:

What are we going to do about my failing eyesight? During this morning's office visit you demanded we hold all chemotherapy until somebody fixes my eyes. Who will do it? No vision care facility will schedule any procedure of repair until I am done with chemotherapy and disease. You and I both know there is no such date.

My body currently complains of Navelbine and Xeloda saturation, yet my mind believes any interruption of chemicals will allow the cancer to explode. I am in a really big jam. You and I argued this morning. It's been a long time since we argued.

I left your office in a huff and took my place on one of those stained chairs by the back door of the complex. That is where broken bodies await community transit—or the end of their life, whichever comes first. Waiting provided ample time for eyesight dilemma and argument to sink in. I proceeded to ponder. God have mercy.

My decline of vision began last November and worsened at an alarming rate. For five months Neal drove me around seeking help. We conferred with a local ophthalmologist, Florida Eye Institute, Bascom Palmer, a low-vision specialist, the Lions Club, and the National Federation of the Blind. We met ourselves coming and going through these six revolving doors. They all agreed slight cataracts and retina swelling could be corrected if or when I finished treatment and disease. In other words, they all agreed not to touch me with a ten-foot instrument. But that's fine because their uniform diagnosis did not jive. The severe distortion I see is not a typical cataract symptom.

In January, my family snatched my car keys and placed

me on house arrest. They claimed intense love, but stripping away my independence is nothing but sheer punishment.

Let me try to fully explain the blind predicament of your long-time patient. I say *try* because typing this down without the use of occasional profanity seems like an injustice. This latest assault on my body and spirit makes me downright furious. I would be dishonest to indicate otherwise. Nothing quite raises the volume of *furious* like sailor language…however…since you think of me as a lady, a good Christian lady, and as I have never wanted to disappoint a teacher or a parent or an imaginary big brother, I will pick and choose my verbiage carefully. So, are we good to go? Are you ready? (One of my favorite questions for the doctor is *are you ready?*)

With driving privileges revoked, I must schedule, at least a week in advance, willing participants to drive me to town for shopping, doctor's appointments, tests, errands, church events, you name it.

Those who get stuck with shopping duty must also take control of the list, maneuver the cart, and choose the groceries, gifts, cards, drugs, clothes, or personal items because I cannot see what freaking aisle I need to be in or what the heck I'm looking for. If there are any embarrassing items on the shopping list, and I don't know that day's driver very well, I have to find the list, find the fat black marker, find the stupid item on the list by way of magnifying glass, and strike it out before he/she gets to my front door. The unmentionable item then gets erased from my mind and consequently, is never purchased. But my chemo brain can't remember why I needed it in the first place so it all comes out in the wash.

Back to blindness. People who transport me hover, breathe down my neck, guide me by the arm, and point out curbs, steps, rough terrain, bright yellow cement parking blocks, steel poles, or innocent people standing nearby and, regardless of warnings, I still manage an incident or two. My sister will tell you—I am a bad girl. One day I planned an escape from her hovering by driving a cart very fast through

Wal-mart's Christmas section. I rammed into an end display causing a ceramic angel to fall off the top shelf, breaking her face and wings. Everyone at the nearby checkout uttered in unison "Oooohhh!"

Connie Titus can no longer be trusted to enter the *proper* public restroom alone, and someone must monitor zippers, skirt hems, and streams of toilet paper that may possibly be attached to my shoes.

What happens during house arrest? First I'll tell you what doesn't happen during house arrest. Thank God there are no bathroom monitors and I can still shower and dress myself. Tee shirts may be worn backwards or inside out, but I am covered.

There is no reading, no writing, or arithmetic. No TV. All television programs or movies resemble *Star Wars'* bar scenes.[72] People have four gross eyeballs across their foreheads, ears on cheeks, and their white, collared shirts shoot upwards, slicing their heads in two. Bodies are sheer. I can see bookcases or doorjambs right through them.

No one wants to engage me in a phone conversation because I do not talk or think positive. Music makes me cry. Kitchen work burns, breaks, or spills. Organizing incoming mail, reading recipes, or looking up important phone numbers with a magnifying glass gives me a headache.

Worst of all, my love of writing has died. You, Doc, have been one of my biggest cheerleaders in this department. Well, drop your pompom. Last Thursday, while cursing and crying, I packed up everything I ever wrote and shoved it into our attic. My theory is if it's not lying around in plain sight, I can't mourn the loss. Cute pun, huh? Plain sight.

Neal reads greeting cards and emails to me in the evenings although his fingers do not know how to respond. Occasionally I meander into the computer room, click reply, type a blind answer to someone's message, hit send, and just hope it goes to the right person. Recipients do forgive my typographical errors, for which I am thankful.

For me to type a letter or greeting such as this, my nose needs to practically touch the computer screen. I enlarge the font to twenty-two points or larger with bold and double space features. When the piece is complete, I magnify the screen 150%—but in order to see a complete line, I would need a monitor as big as a picture window. As is, I can only look at and make corrections to the left side of the sentence, then the middle, then the right side, line by line. Hours later, if all appears flawless to the blind woman, I return the document to a normal font and format, and print it out for Neal's proofreading. Drat. Even thinking about this long, drawn-out process zaps my will to continue.

What is God thinking—allowing loss after loss? He only hurts himself. I cannot drive myself down avenues of ministry delivering baked goods or devotions to the sick or lonely. What better way to serve him? There are no more meetings with the Lord of the Dance at his sanctuary on the beach. The ocean was my best place to enjoy him. I cannot read God's Holy Word. Reading the Bible was a sure way to believe in him and find direction, for Christ's sake! Singing hymns of praise or playing "How Great Thou Art" [73] on the clarinet doesn't work if I can't see the music. But this pleased him so. Writing down all of God's miracles in my life is supposed to further his kingdom, not cause me anguish! These activities are gifts from him, but without clear eyesight, it all comes to a screeching halt. Did he slap me in the face? Feels like it.

After the slap came deep depression and I dragged the family down with me. What is a woman's purpose if she's blind as a bat? In early days of marriage, Neal used to kid around and refer to me as the old bat. Now I am the blind old bat. Seriously, without my eyesight, what good am I? Our very first grandchild is due in February. At this rate I'll only be able to smell him or her.

House arrest activities were reduced to hand watering the lawn or garden for hours and lying still on the couch or bed for hours, day after day, with a blank stare. I didn't even care to pray.

Acceptance followed depression, though, thank God. There's been no improvement, mind you. Vision today measures 20/200 [L], 20/400 [R]. My eyes are what they are. I am not going to spend any more time or money trying to figure it out. God will help me find a way around this, but I wish he would snap to it. I love J. Ellsworth Kalas' frank talk. "If God wants to do a good thing for us, why can't he do it now?"[74]

Here we are, at present time. Pondering ends.

All kinds of patients and attitudes sit on the stained chairs by the back door of your medical complex—waiting, thinking. Moods happen, choices are made. Each chaired participant handles hard knocks their own way. The middle-aged grow older while the young-at-heart make plans; the depressed want to chuck it all, but dreamers travel the world over; angry people curse while sitting next to survivors giving thanks. (I can be every one of the above.) White blood cells respond accordingly.

After walking out of your office this morning, I proceeded to destroy my mood until a handsome, healthy gentleman sat down beside me. He said he needed to retreat from the air conditioning for a few moments of warmth. His voice and scent and character resembled you, my friend. But why would a white-coated professional sit on a dirty chair next to the back door, conversing with a somewhat gray lady whom he just argued with? My eyes fail. Were you real or imagined?

You were real. A visual conversation started with digital camera in hand. Your colorful travelogue scooped me off to Scotland, to New York, to the mountains. Together we viewed images of blue-plaid kilts (with or without bare knees or *whatever*), a family gathered around a Seder meal, and a cashmere bride accompanying her man on a shopping spree for a new piano. Frolic and laughter broke loose like you and I were best friends again. In a few moments time, my attitude turned upward and your chilled body warmed. I bet if Nurse

Molly checked our white counts, we would both register nice and plenty.

Just then my favorite gray-bearded chauffeur arrived. He shook your hand and hugged my neck, uttering an observation. "Hmmm. The last time I came to collect you at the doctor's office, this same gentleman sat next to you in the chemo room, holding your hand. He must love you very much."

Yes, it is true. He must love me very much.

Thank you for the most memorable Tuesday yet. Thank you for being real.

Love,

Connie

Connie Titus (blind as a bat but making plans, traveling the world over, and giving thanks with nice and plenty white blood cells).

Wednesday, May 23, 2007

Good Evening, Dr. Collin, Long-Time Friend:

In the tenth year, in the third month, on the twenty-third day, I muse over the number of times you and I escorted each other in and out of exam rooms, classrooms, and concert halls and how your curved forefinger pointed the way—to nowhere on occasion—but at least you cared enough to stick your neck out and direct. I maneuvered you too, by sharpening your sensitivities, breaking down your emotional barriers, and training you to land on both feet with a smile. The score may be tied, except I never sent you a bill.

We still walk clinic hallways together, but have you noticed? I've not written a letter to you for nine months. Are you relieved or concerned? A phenomenal gestation period of miracles has just taken place. I am still trying to figure out how or why I am worthy of these miracles. Oh, what God has done for me! I scarce can take it in. "…they cannot fathom what God has done from beginning to end" (Ecclesiastes 3:11, NIV).

And the Lord's calendar, his timepiece is awesome. "He has made everything beautiful in its time" (Ecclesiastes 3:11, NIV).

Why *does* God do what he does, and when? "…God does it so that men will revere him" (Ecclesiastes 3:14, NIV). Ezekiel expands on why God does it—so they, and you and I, and we all will know that God is God. As for me and my household, *we believe!* I offer my reverence and respect for this awesome God in one last letter to you. Stand beside me, Dr. Collin. Stand right here beside me.

• • •

"…a time to scatter stones and a time to gather them…"
(Ecclesiastes 3:5, NIV).

This reminds me of the diseased lymph nodes in my neck

and chest. They scatter for awhile, then they gather themselves to pester me. You warned me my disease would keep popping up, and so it does, like pop-up blockers on the computer—*bloop, bloop, bloop*. And when the warning pops up, we hit the Red X to minimize. Is there a ready supply of Red X in your closet? I've moved from drug to drug to drug since November 2005. *Red X* Navelbine/Xeloda followed by *Red X* Taxol/Carboplatin were not much fun. Now we select another *Red X*, Gemzar, leading me into a weekly meeting with you and your pop-up blocker squad. By the way, I am grateful you and your squad have not tired, scattered, or run off thus far. Thank you.

Divine Intervention lends favor despite pop-up warnings. Let us raise a toast to God. Lymph nodes with continual disease usually transmit bad cells everywhere. As I write this letter, there is no organ or bone involvement in the body of Connie Titus. Talk about reverence...is this another miracle, or what? "...And then you will know that I am the Lord" (Ezekiel 13:23, NIV).

I am mindful that without *bloop, bloop, bloop*, and without the assistance (or the endurance) of your *Red X*, God wouldn't need to perform miracles for me; my current ministry to others wouldn't exist. So it is possible to catch a glimpse of a purpose for trial and tribulation...a purpose for scattering and gathering. Good reasons to press ahead.

• • •

"...a time to keep, and a time to cast away..."
(Ecclesiastes 3:6, KJV).

"... and a time to laugh ..." (Ecclesiastes 3:4, NIV).

Even in current treatment, I envision the ten years, three months, twenty-three days of cancer as an isolated season. I cast it away, behind me, far, far away. Building my future is entirely possible.

Fifteen years down the road, when you are age seventy-two and I am a mere sixty-eight, I will come collect you on a

Tuesday afternoon for a leisurely drive in the country. We'll take my dark green Malibu. I will drive. To answer your earlier question, no, the Malibu is not a convertible; however, I have fifteen years to make it so, and there is something about you that empowers me to saw the hardtop off all by myself. And when we are stopped for speeding on Route 66 (like Vonnie's husband), I will look pitiful, inform the officer I suffer from cancer (an arrest of any kind is definitely a time to keep cancer), and introduce you as my aged oncologist, explaining that in our combined deteriorating condition, we must get to every destination *fast*. But where is our destination, do you know? Was it ice cream or sea mist? At any rate, laughing puts zest in them dry bones and God allots time for laughing. Yes, my Lord endorses laughter.

• • •

"…a time to be born…" (Ecclesiastes 3:2, NIV).

Behold a wondrous story concerning a time to be born. First, let me set the stage.

Cancer survivorship begins with a date on the calendar, a diagnosis date. Last November I conducted a case study among peers, asking how they felt about their diagnosis dates. Look what I found.

Fifty-five percent of survivors nestle the day of shocking news and, when it comes time, they pull up the details and retreat to the closet for a good, loud cry. But these folks emerge refreshed, ready to go at life some more. Ten percent curse or kick around their ugly day (bad deal). Each year their bitterness increases. Another ten percent seal diagnoses dates into Ziploc bags and send them to the unconscious part of the brain where misery is simply forgotten. My husband and children are members of the Ziploc crowd. They would rather not be reminded.

I, on the other hand, along with the remaining twenty-five percent, embrace and accept my diagnosis date with a lively, determined spirit. I choose to treat the day as my *birth-*

day because each year the miracle of survival is magnified. The Lord presents me with birthday gifts and you've read about them in previous pages. Survival is truly good reason to marvel and celebrate.

I exchange humorous birthday cards with one friend whose diagnosis is the same month, same year. Our husbands roll their eyes. Several years ago I got all gussied up and invited Neal out for a fancy candlelight dinner. He asked me what the occasion was. I smiled. "It's my birthday."

"No, it's not," he argued. "I may be getting senile, but today is not your birthday."

I explained.

"Oh, that." My dear husband's eyes drooped into a sad shade of blue and he no longer enjoyed his meal. But that did not stop me. I kept smiling, bouncing to the music, savoring every breath and bite.

Wednesday, January 24, 2007, was my tenth birthday, the tenth anniversary of my diagnosis. A little boy child was born that evening. I was sick that day and had to wear a blue mask to protect myself and those around me, but this little boy child recognized me anyway because my blood runs through his veins. His name is Alexander Enrique Gonzalez, and he is my very first grandchild.

Listen to the amazing part of this story: Alexander Enrique Gonzalez came to us nineteen days early due to mommy's complications. Tuesday, January 23, a nurse wheeled our daughter Caryn into the hospital for inducement of labor. Induction drugs don't always produce immediate results. Baby Alex could have been born that day, or stretched his birthday out to Thursday, January 25, or gone full-term, entering the world on Monday, February 12. No. Thoughtful God picked Wednesday, January 24. And God's perfect hour chimed at 7:23 p.m. while a chancel choir harmonized and prayed in a familiar sanctuary. This beloved group has long been in tune with our family's physical, emotional, and spiritual cycles.

Who can deny the Creator of all mankind implements

sweet timing? Oh, the reward of life and reason for my striving. I have just been blessed with the brightest birthday gift of all, and how gently God placed him in my arms.

Doctor Collin, friend, my blood runs through your veins, too. One day Caryn and I placed my birthday bundle of baby into *your* arms. Nurses and staff formed a long line in the hallway, receiving him beautifully. Alex was a hands-on thank-you card for ushering our family to this miracle milestone. God spoke up in all his glory, "… and you will know that I am the Lord" (Ezekiel 16:62, NIV).

Sometimes he causes me to tremble…tremble…tremble.

• • •

"…and a time to heal…" (Ecclesiastes 3:3, NIV).

After eighteen months of blindness and especially missing out on our firstborn grandson's facial expressions, Neal and I checked in with one of the vision care facilities. All I meant to do was draw diagrams of my visual distortion. Florida Eye Institute's female ophthalmologist threw her hands up, proclaimed huge cataracts, suggested surgery would restore my eyesight 90-100%, and asked what in the world I was waiting for. Florida Eye Institute's male retinal specialist disagreed. He said my cataracts were only moderate, surgery may or may not fix me, but one cataract must be removed for a clear view into other issues.

God's Institute said it was time for Connie Titus' eyes to be healed. Surgeries were scheduled and conducted May 2 and May 9.

When the first surgical bandage was removed, that eye could see near perfect. All the way home I read detailed billboards and license plates to my sister. We both cried. Second surgery proved even better results than the first. Institute doctors surprised themselves. I loved your cute comment yesterday, thanking God for a woman surgeon who had the *balls* to get in there and get the job done. And to that I added "Amen, brother!"

This little boy child, Alexander, and I are linked together with our big brown eyes. As his infant eyes focus for the first time on color, texture, and movement, I experience the same pleasure. While Alex gets tickled about the ceiling fan (moving or not), his Daddy's red bath towel, and the workings of his own little feet and toes, I marvel over glistening blades of grass and strands of hair blowing in the wind—not my hair, or Neal's, not yours or the Pastor's, since we are all bald, but there *are* people with strands of hair blowing in the wind. I've seen it with my own eyes.

At last, car keys jingle in my hand. Let freedom ring. I am the only woman in town who smiles and waves at speed limit signs.

Yes, Baby Alex and Grandma Connie's big brown eyes drink in everything God has to offer and he repeatedly announces, "Then you will know that I am the Lord, your God" (Ezekiel 20:20, NIV). Dr. Collin, make note of quoted verse 20:20. Perfect vision is spelled out.

• • •

"...a time to be silent and a time to speak..."
(Ecclesiastes 3:7, NIV).

Eighteen months of blindness was a time for silence. But the day the second surgical bandage was removed—that very afternoon—I received a phone message from a publisher interested in a manuscript I put together back in 2005. (Oh boy, oh boy—a time to see *and* speak.) What is the manuscript about? Are you ready for this? My manuscript is a compilation of the letters in your citrus box. Do you have any objections to our relationship being read by the public?

The publisher's contract, a red and yellow package, lay like a gem on my garage floor. My restored eyesight feasted on every word of opportunity. I signed, sealed, and delivered that offer yesterday, Tuesday morning, May 22, 2007. Silence gives way to my voice in print. Maybe you and I can be a sign together. Other doctor-patient teams could view our shining example, learn to smile at one another, cut each other some slack, and roll up their sleeves for a common purpose. You have encouraged me for years, with my writing. We shall see what God does with this. "…you will speak…and will no longer be silent. So you [Connie Titus and Alan S. Collin, M.D.] will be a sign to them, and they will know that I am the Lord" (Ezekiel 24:27, NIV).

• • •

"…a time to dance…" (Ecclesiastes 3:4, NIV).

"You turned my wailing into dancing; you removed my sackcloth and clothed me with joy, that my heart may sing to you…O Lord my God…" (Psalm 30:11-12, NIV).

Our doctor-patient success culminates, my good man, and the harvest of your goofy prescription to dance at daybreak is my elongated strength and a whole new way of life. Our musical score wraps around years of harmony and instruction and seems complete at this point. And I believe, if you want to get technical about it, you and I are two changed people.

But a majestic symphony is rarely the end of a story. I must dance a while longer.

It is 5:10 a.m. I have just finished this epistle during my Tuesday-can't-sleep-all-night steroid buzz. My sweet daughter and family sleep soundly in the guest room. Excuse me now. I will awaken Baby Alexander. He and I will sneak out together and drive up over a tall bridge toward sunrise. I will lift my short, very handsome dance partner high for a blessing at the surf's edge, then we will twirl and boogey in the sand just as you prescribed.

In one of my letters I talked about how love is the answer—for life, for health and peace. A child's love pours out so sweet, so pure. Baby Alex doesn't mind if I wake him up out of a sound sleep. It's okay with him if I'm flat on one side. Alexander Enrique Gonzalez recognizes and accepts me in a blue mask, an ugly compression sleeve, a red ball cap, a psychedelic bandana covered with peace signs, a blond or brunette wig, or a soft covering of gray peach fuzz. I am his favorite any time, any how, any place or way. Truly, truly I say to you: Love is the answer.

My life begins all over again. "Then sings my soul, my Savior God to thee. How great thou art."[75]

Dr. Alan S. Collin, you've been so intimately involved in my journey hitherto. God and you turned my wailing into dancing. The two of you removed my sackcloth and clothed me with joy (and some blue paper on Tuesdays). Join us for the sequel of my life. Are you ready, my friend? Here we go, here we go!

May peace and grace be yours,

Connie

Connie Beth Thompson Titus

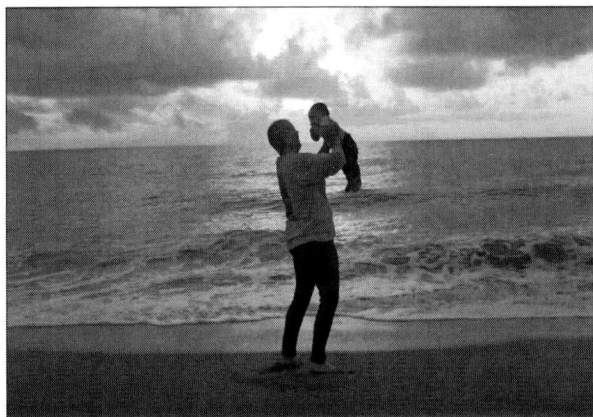

"Children's children are a crown to the aged..." (Proverbs 17:6, NIV). "Praise the Lord. Sing to the Lord a new song..." (Psalm 149:1, NIV). "Let them praise his name with dancing and make music to him..." (Psalm 149:3, NIV). In the land of beginning again, dreams come true. Prayers are in reach of the Ocean Maker.

Courtesy of Photographer Caryn Gonzalez

Acknowledgements

A creative writer takes shape by listening to and watching folks from his or her path. And insistent friends persuade a novice author to come out of the closet. I win because my whole community of influence is a happy, positive crowd. They are the reason I accomplish this writing project with joy. I pay tribute to them.

First award goes to our Father who art in heaven. He organizes dear people along my path, he sustains my living, and he directs my gift. Words occasionally run together on the pages and I can't remember what I ate for breakfast, but the Lord empowers me to complete this composition with focus and determination. *Thank you, Lord God Almighty. I feel your guidance and blessing even amidst frank, blatant talk. And I am so grateful you lead me into a dance, wherever I may be. I pray my artistry and my dance steps bring you glory.*

Second honorable mention goes to my sweet husband who sits quietly alone in front of the television, attempts to play musical duets by himself, or cuddles with a pillow in an empty bed while my fingers peck away at the keyboard. He believes in me and reads my work with enthusiasm. *Neal, your patience enables my creativity to flow. I adore you.*

Hale, hearty, and charming children capture my healing on film, roll out the red carpet for letter writing, and bring my survival goals into reach. *Caryn, Ron, Jaime, and Alexander, your surprises, your cheerleading, your love for me and one another gives me the green light to live, live, and live some more. Thank you.*

Loving family members, friends, co-workers, medical personnel, and cancer buddies read pieces of my raw talent and suggest I go to print. *You honor me. Published authors must first know what a dangling participle is—which I do not—but you honor me.* [Smile]

Hebrew prophets of old, psalmists, and disciples of a Resurrected Man have penned and preserved amazing truths that transfer my stance with cancer from sinking sand to solid ground. *Your holy penmanship imparts our Lord's spirit and character until I crave him all the more. I would surely like to shake your hands in person one day.*

Authors, singers, and songwriters everywhere identify my psyche as if they are peeking through my window. *Thanks for allowing what I read, hear, and understand in your work to spill over into my work. I hereby applaud two spiritual heroes, Rabbi Lawrence A. Hoffman and Dr. J. Ellsworth Kalas.*

A young lady in a church sound booth keeps me current and accountable with no editing or constructive criticism in mind. Two new friends pick up where she leaves off. *Jean, Betty, and Connie, the stimulating support you offer is extra and oh, so motivating. Many thanks for ushering me into publication.*

What professional photographer, in his right mind, says "yes" to a photo session inside a cancer clinic? *Jerry Brewer, Photographer Extraordinaire, your portraits of truth and humor say it all, just as I had hoped. I appreciate your bravery. Great job, buddy!*

Courageous ophthalmologist Dr. Karen Todd is kind enough to get in there and repair my eyeballs so I can graciously accept a lovely invitation from Stacy, Jesika, Lindsay, Amanda, Kandi, Stefanie and Faith of Tate Publishing. *Beautiful women stand in my corner. Thank you all for assisting God with my healing and speaking.*

Finally, a heap of gratitude pours out to the licensed professional himself, Alan S. Collin, M.D. *Without your antics these pages would be blank, my dancing shoes stuck in the back of the closet, and my bones dry. What robust subject matter you are. Take everything I've written as a compliment. I tip my hat to you.*

101 Coping Ideas
(In No Particular Order)

"Each one should use whatever gift he has received to serve others, faithfully administering God's grace in its various forms" (1 Peter 4:10, NIV). "What a wonderful God we have—the One who comforts us in our hardships and trials. And why does he do this? So that when others are troubled, needing our sympathy and encouragement, we can pass on to them this same help and comfort God has given us" (2 Corinthians 1:3-4, TLB).

God gave me the gift of writing and he offered me great comfort during hardships and trials; therefore, I must pass on the same help and comfort he lavished on me. People ask what I do to keep going. Below are 101 things I do, think, and believe that keep me in forward motion. Diagnoses, treatments, and lifestyles may differ, but many of my suggestions work for any illness. A word of caution: well-meaning people can overwhelm you with tips (like me). You have no obligation. Use your instincts. Pick and choose.

• • •

Please consider…

1. doing what is in your power to help yourself.[76]

2. that "life is worth living, people are worth loving, and God is worth trusting." (Author unknown).

3. lying on the couch like a slug, without guilt.

4. journaling, keeping a diary.

5. listing short-term and long-term goals, referring to them often.

6. discovering your own secret to life and living.

7. picturing Jesus with one hand on the chemo pole or radiation machine and one hand on your shoulder, singing a hymn with you, harmonizing.

8. pushing yourself when you don't feel like it, stretching beyond belief, reaching for the sun and the Son.

9. working during treatment, or not—jobs provide purpose and diversion, yet public contact becomes risky with low blood counts. Talk it over with your family and your doctor.

10. making friends with Bernie S. Siegel, M.D. (*Love, Medicine and Miracles*), [77] and Andrew Weil, M.D. (*Eight Weeks to Optimum Health*) [78] —authors of mind/body communication.

11. that people want to help, it makes them feel good. Jot down ingredients for your favorite casserole to give to well-meaning cooks.

12. a low-impact aerobic video or DVD.

13. total body massage and reflexology.

14. sensitivity to the fullness of life.[79]

15. drinking six to eight 8-oz. glasses of distilled water a day, green tea, and 100% fruit juice in lieu of sodas.

16. dynamic imagery, vivid positive imagination, and visualization.

17. using deodorant instead of antiperspirant.

18. maneuvering a new look—painting expressive eye makeup; wearing unusual earrings; trying wigs of all colors, lengths, and styles; changing turbans, hats, and scarves as your mood strikes (men, pass on this—bald is sexy enough, no baubles, bangles or beads needed).

19. checking into vitamins, supplements, herbal remedies (after chemo).

20. cleaning closets, starting household projects even if you can't finish.

21. that being "one with God is a majority."[80]

22. playing a game with bald heads, rubbing them for good fortune, and following Dave Dravecky's suggestion to scare away unwanted door-to-door salesmen.

23. the healing rewards of praying for others, and please know that praying for yourself is *not* selfish.

24. trying the Highland Fling by a treehouse, a flash dance in an exam room, and the samba out by the seashore when the sun comes up.

25. listening to your body and accepting its thorn(s).

• • •

I endorse...

26. fantasy.

27. reality.

28. eating six small meals a day.

29. beginner line-dancing classes, but only to music of the '70s.

30. a mild sedative.

31. old movies, sad or funny.

32. acting ridiculous—any behavior is appropriate.

33. opening up communication lines, relishing intimacy, and telling folks what hurts.

34. the soothing properties of hot showers.

35. chasing rainbows (*respectable, true colors*).

36. antioxidants, but not during chemotherapy.

37. music, all kinds, *your* favorites—not the family favorites.

38. a *Patch Adams* oncologist or primary care physician, one who is top-notch in his field but knows how to be silly.

39. simplifying the home, ridding your cubbyhole and mind of clutter.

40. echinacea, garlic, crystallized ginger, evening primrose oil, and flaxseed oil.

41. a walk on the beach at sunrise, at sunset, in the moonlight.

42. relaxation, whatever that is.

43. talking with old people who have been through it all, twice, uphill, both ways.

44. The Hokey-Pokey, the Mazurka, and even a good box-step (any time of day).

45. writing a letter of dismay, handing it to the postman or not.

46. letting others make decisions.

47. natural, organic, fresh everything.

48. staying up late and sleeping late.

49. singing, dancing, and playing an instrument—in key, in sync, or otherwise.

50. Paint by Number, Twister, and Duck Duck Goose.

• • •

By all means…

51. ask questions.

52. watch for angels inside ordinary people.

53. scream into a pillow, dig a deep hole in the back yard, bury the pillow, wave and smile at gawking neighbors.

54. maintain hobbies and interests, or start something new.

55. stock ice cream.

56. get down on the floor with your pets, your children, or grandchildren—become like them.

57. believe in your decisions.

58. laugh often, invite comedians into your living room on a daily basis.

59. go outdoors, stand amidst nature fifteen minutes a day, and walk to the mailbox.

60. screen your calls, stand over the answer machine while it's still talking, take three to four weeks to return calls.

61. dance with the real Lord of the Dance.

62. read, read, read; study medications, dosages, side effects; attend support groups.

63. monitor your stress level.

64. plant, weed, dig, and sweat in the garden.

65. let it all hang out, cry all you want—it's your party.

66. use the best of both worlds—orthodox and alternative.

67. while you wait in a checkout line, break into the Twist or the Jitterbug. Offer a candy bar to anyone who joins you.

68. get mad, work up some determination, and argue with God. Moses did. And Dr. Kalas says it is all right to argue with God. "I am very grateful, O God, that you will allow me to argue with you, even when I know you will win."[81]

69. do a naked rain dance.

70. look under every rock for a cure.

71. hire it done.

72. stay in your pajamas all day long.

73. treat this difficult season like a new adventure.

74. seek the company of supportive, positive family members and friends—run from the grumps.

75. take control of the remote.

• • •

Remember...

76. you are never too old for teddy bears or blankies.

77. whole grains are best (try Ezekiel Sesame Bread).

78. to pack a goody bag for the chemo room: favorite craft, magazine, comic book, comfort foods and drinks (no alcohol, please).

79. that wearing purple and/or red makes a statement you are alive and vibrant.

80. God is ever ready by your side to provide physical rest and awareness, deepen his relationship with you, and deliver spiritual nourishment to you and your caregivers.

81. to eat a nutritious, healthy pyramid. More fruits and vegetables. More fish and chicken.

82. don't be afraid to tell people you want to be alone.

83. don't be afraid to invite sixty-one people to come by.

84. dark chocolate.

85. to load up your grocery cart with anti-cancer foods (as stated in Letter #44).

86. God never sleeps and he never slumbers. Read Psalm 121:3.

87. doctors are informed practitioners available to assist, but they do not know it all, they do not decide how an illness will or will not progress, and they cannot control attitudes.

88. deep breathing clean air in through the nose and out through the mouth.

89. to read labels.

90. to steer clear of pesticides, insecticides, and cleaning agent fumes—investigate natural products that can accomplish the job.

91. God can deliver us all through dark, winding tunnels…if only we ask.

92. to open the best manual available—the Holy Bible.

93. occasional beer, wine, or blackberry brandy hit the spot.

94. God works through authors. He knows what you need to read and when. Seek a daily devotion book.

95. zest for life, vigor, taking hold, and holding fast, and if you're happy and you know it, notify your face.

96. Robert Fulghum is right: warm cookies and cold milk are good for you.

97. when the Lifeguard Station sign says *Keep Off,* it does not apply to cancer patients. We can do as we please.

98. don't get too big for your britches. Get down off your high horse, but get back up on your high horse, as needed.

99. to sleep in total darkness.

100. God's "…saving power will rise on you like the sun and bring healing like the sun's rays" (Malachi 4:2, GNT). What a fabulous reason to dance, dance, dance at daybreak.

• • •

I pray for…

101. the freedom of your dancing heart.

Notes to the Text

1 Linda Ronstadt, "I've Got a Crush on You" (Los Angeles: Elektra/Asylum Label, 1983).

2 *Lost in Space* (Los Angeles: Twentieth Century Fox Studios, 1965), Director Alvin Ganzer; Actor Bill Mumy.

3 *Under The Tuscan Sun* (Burbank, CA: Walt Disney Video Studio, 2003), Director Audrey Wells; Actress Diane Lane.

4 Earth, Wind & Fire, "Celebrate" (New York: Sony Label, 1975).

5 Earth, Wind & Fire, "I'll Write a Song for You" (Miami, FL: Pyramid Records Corp., 1996).

6 Susun S. Weed, *Breast Cancer? Breast Health! The Wise Woman* Way (New York: Ash Tree Publishing, 1996), 150.

7 Earth, Wind & Fire, "Let's Groove" (Miami, FL: Pyramid Records Corp., 1996).

8 Earth, Wind & Fire, "Be Ever Wonderful" (Miami, FL: Pyramid Records Corp., 1996).

9 *Mad About You* (Culver City, CA: Sony Pictures Studio, 1992), Director Linda Day; Actress Helen Hunt.

10 *The Wizard of Oz* (Burbank, CA: Warner Bros., 1939), Director Victor Fleming; Actress Judy Garland.

11 Susan M. Love, M.D., *Dr. Susan Love's Breast Book* (Massachusetts: Addison-Wesley Publishing Company, 1995), 342.

12 The Benedictine Monks of Santo Domingo De Silos, "Gregorian Chant" (Madrid: Angel Records Label, 1994).

13 William Shakespeare, *The Tempest* (UK: Ginn & Company, 1888), 39.

14 Mrs. Charles Cowman, *Streams in the Desert, Anniversary Edition* (Michigan: The Zondervan Corporation, 1996), 373-374.

15 Earth, Wind & Fire, "Sing a Song" (Miami, FL: Pyramid Records Corp., 1996).

16 *Billy Joel Easy Piano Collection* (Milwaukee, WI: Hal Leonard Corporation, 1987).

17 *Garfield* Greeting Card (Indiana: Paws, Inc., 1978), Cartoonist Jim Davis.

18 Earth, Wind & Fire, "Mighty Might" (New York: Sony Label, 1974).

19 Helen Reddy, "You and Me Against the World" (Hollywood, CA: Capitol Records Label, 1975).

20 *Look Good, Feel Better Program,* (Washington, D.C.: CTFA Foundation; Atlanta, GA: American Cancer Society, 1993), www.lookgoodfeelbetter.org.

21 Earth, Wind & Fire, "Let Your Feelings Show" (Miami, FL: Pyramid Records Corp., 1996).

22 Charles F. Stanley (Atlanta, GA: In Touch Ministries, Inc., 1982).

23 *A Christmas Story* (Burbank, CA: Warner Bros., 1983), Director Bob Clark; Actor Darren McGavin.

24 Earth, Wind & Fire, "Fantasy" (Miami, FL: Pyramid Records Corp., 1996).

25 *High Anxiety* (Los Angeles, CA: Twentieth Century Fox Studios, 1977), Director Mel Brooks; Actor Mel Brooks.

26 Robert Fulghum, *All I Really Need To Know I Learned in Kindergarten* (New York: Ballantine Books, 1988).

27 J. Ellsworth Kalas, *The Grand Sweep: 365 Days from Genesis through Revelation* (Tennessee: Abingdon Press, 1996), 213.

28 Frank Sinatra, "Softly As I Leave You" (Burbank, CA: Warner Bros. Records, Inc., 1968).

29 J. Ellsworth Kalas, *The Grand Sweep: 365 Days from Genesis through Revelation* (Tennessee: Abingdon Press, 1996), 105.

30 J. Ellsworth Kalas, *The Grand Sweep: 365 Days from Genesis through Revelation* (Tennessee: Abingdon Press, 1996), 152.

31 *Fatal Attraction* (Hollywood, CA: Paramount Studio, 1987), Director Adrian Lyne; Actor Michael Douglas.

32 J. Ellsworth Kalas, *The Grand Sweep: 365 Days from Genesis through Revelation* (Tennessee: Abingdon Press, 1996), 207.

33 Bill Withers, "Lean on Me" (New York: Sony Label, 1994).

34 "I Believe" (New York: Cromwell Music, Inc., 1952), words and music by Ervin Drake, Irvin Graham, Jimmy Shirl and Al Stillman.

35 *Fiddler on the Roof* (Los Angeles, CA: MGM Studio, 1971), Director Norman Jewison; Actor Topol.

36 *Patch Adams* (Hollywood, CA: Universal Studios, 1998), Director Tom Shadvac; Actor Robin Williams.

37 *Deep Impact* (Hollywood, CA: Paramount Studio, 1998), Director Mimi Leder; Actor Maximilian Schell.

38 *Chemotherapy and You* (Bethesda, MD: National Cancer Institute, National Institute of Health, 1996).

39 Dave Dravecky, Jan Dravecky and Joni Eareckson Tada, ed., *NIV Encouragement Bible* (Michigan: Zondervan Publishing House, 2001), 1306.

40 Earth, Wind & Fire, "Shining Star" (Miami, FL: Pyramid Records Corp., 1996).

41 *Nicole Johnson Live: Stepping into the Ring* (Santa Monica, CA: Fresh Brewed Life, Inc., 2002), www.freshbrewedlife. com.

42 Earth, Wind & Fire, "That's the Way of the World" (Miami, FL: Pyramids Records Corp., 1996).

43 Anonymous.

44 England Dan and John Ford Coley, "Love is the Answer" (New York: Rhino/Wea Label, 1976).

45 *Art.Rage.Us.* (San Francisco, CA: Chronicle Books, 1998).

46 Robert Louis Stevenson, *The Silverado Squatters* (London: Chatto & Windus, 1883).

47 Diana Krall, "When I Look in Your Eyes" (New York: Avatar Studios, Verve Label, 1999), Lyricist Leslie Bricusse.

48 The Canadian Brass, "Concierto de Aranjuez" (New York: Soundtrack Studio A, 1995).

49 The Moody Blues, "Forever Afternoon (Tuesday?)" (UK: Polydor/umgd Label, 1967).

50 Ray Bradbury as quoted by Kay Minto, *Art.Rage.Us.* (San Francisco: Chronicle Books, 1998), 124.

51 "It Is Well With My Soul," words by Horatio G. Spafford, 1873; music by Philip P. Bliss, 1876.

52 *The Passion of the Christ* (Los Angeles, CA: Twentieth Century Fox Studio, 2004), Director Mel Gibson; Actor James Caviezel.

53 Temptations, "Night and Day," Soundtrack for *What Women Want* (New York: Sony Label, 2000).

54 Rabbi Morris N. Kertzer and Rabbi Lawrence A. Hoffman, *What is a Jew?* (New York: Touchstone—Simon & Schuster, Inc., 1993), excerpts xix-281.

55 *The Book of Worship for Church and Home* (Tennessee: The Methodist Publishing House, 1965).

56 Ruth Rosen, ed., *Jewish Doctors Meet the Great Physician* (San Francisco: Purple Pomegranate Productions, 1998), 16.

57 "Here I Am, Lord," words and music by Dan Schutte, 1981.

58 Neil Diamond, "Hello Again" (New York: Sony Label, 1982).

59 Olivia Newton-John, "I Honestly Love You" (UK: EMI Label, 1974).

60 *Apollo* 13 (Hollywood, CA: Universal Studios, 1995), Director Ron Howard; Actor Tom Hanks.

61 Ralph Waldo Emerson, *The Complete Sermons of Ralph Waldo Emerson* (Missouri: University of Missouri Press, 1989), 139.

62 *The Doctor* (Burbank, CA: Walt Disney Studio, 1991), Director Randa Haines; Actor William Hurt.

63 *True Lies* (Los Angeles, CA: Twentieth Century Fox Studios, 1994), Director James Cameron; Actress Jamie Lee Curtis.

64 Joni Eareckson Tada, Dave Dravecky and Jan Dravecky, ed., *NIV Encouragement Bible* (Michigan: Zondervan Publishing House, 2001), 589.

65 Samuel Barber, "Adagio for Strings" (New York: Sony Label, 1969).

66 Earth, Wind & Fire, "That's the Way of the World" (Miami, Florida: Pyramid Records Corp., 1996).

67 James Ingram, "How Do You Keep The Music Playing?" (New York: Warner/Wea Label, 1991).

68 Peobo Bryson, "Silent Night" (New York: Sony Label, 1995).

69 J. Ellsworth Kalas, *The Grand Sweep: 365 Days from Genesis through Revelation* (Tennessee: Abingdon Press, 1996), 229.

70 Earth, Wind & Fire, "That's the Way of the World" (Miami, FL: Pyramid Records Corp., 1996).

71 *The Cosby Show* (Los Angeles, CA: Urban Works Studio, 1984), Director Nancy Stern; Actor Bill Cosby.

72 *Star Wars* (Los Angeles, CA: Twentieth Century Fox Studios, 1980), Director George Lucas; Actress Carrie Fisher.

73 "How Great Thou Art," words and music by Stuart K. Hine, 1953.

74 J. Ellsworth Kalas, *The Grand Sweep: 365 Days from Genesis through Revelation* (Tennessee: Abingdon Press, 1996), 157.

75 "How Great Thou Art," words and Music by Stuart K. Hine, 1953.

76 J. Ellsworth Kalas, *The Grand Sweep: 365 Days from Genesis through Revelation* (Tennessee: Abingdon Press, 1996), 141.

77 Bernie S. Siegel, M.D., *Love, Medicine and Miracles* (New York: HarperCollins Publishers, 1988).

78 Andrew Weil, M.D., *Eight Weeks to Optimum Health* (New York: Ballantine Books, 1998).

79 J. Ellsworth Kalas, *The Grand Sweep: 365 Days from Genesis through Revelation* (Tennessee: Abingdon Press, 1996), 130.

80 J. Ellsworth Kalas, *The Grand Sweep: 365 Days from Genesis through Revelation* (Tennessee: Abingdon Press, 1996), 104.

81 J. Ellsworth Kalas, *The Grand Sweep: 365 Days from Genesis through Revelation* (Tennessee: Abingdon Press, 1996), 153.

Selected Bibliography

Reference to song titles, songwriters, movies, television shows, greeting cards, cancer programs or booklets and books of only incidental reference are not included in this list but are identified in the Notes to the Text.

Bradbury, Ray as quoted by Kay Minto. *Art.Rage.Us.* San Francisco: Chronicle Books, 1998.

Cowman, Mrs. Charles. *Streams in the Desert, Anniversary Edition.* Grand Rapids: The Zondervan Corporation, 1996.

Dravecky, Dave, Jan Dravecky and Joni Eareckson Tada, ed. *NIV Encouragement Bible.* Grand Rapids: The Zondervan Corporation, 2001.

Kalas, J. Ellsworth. *The Grand Sweep: 365 Days from Genesis through Revelation.* Nashville: Abingdon Press, 1996.

Kertzer, Rabbi Morris N., and Rabbi Lawrence A. Hoffman. *What is a Jew?* New York: Touchstone—Simon & Schuster, Inc., 1993.

Love, Susan M., M.D. *Dr. Susan Love's Breast Book.* Reading, Massachusetts: Addison-Wesley Publishing Company, 1995.

Rosen, Ruth, ed. *Jewish Doctors Meet The Great Physician.* San Francisco: Purple Pomegranate Productions, 1998.

Shakespeare, William. *The Tempest.* UK: Ginn & Company, 1888.

Stevenson, Robert Louis. *The Silverado Squatters.* London: Chatto & Windus, 1883.

Tada, Joni Eareckson, Dave Dravecky and Jan Dravecky, ed. *NIV Encouragement Bible*. Grand Rapids: The Zondervan Corporation, 2001.

Weed, Susun S. *Breast Cancer? Breast Health! The Wise Woman Way*. Woodstock, New York: Ash Tree Publishing, 1996.